Pediatric Genetics

Editors

ANNE SLAVOTINEK
BRITTANY SIMPSON
ALLISON TAM

PEDIATRIC CLINICS OF NORTH AMERICA

www.pediatric.theclinics.com

Consulting Editor
TINA L. CHENG

October 2023 • Volume 70 • Number 5

ELSEVIER

1600 John F. Kennedy Boulevard • Suite 1800 • Philadelphia, Pennsylvania, 19103-2899

http://www.theclinics.com

THE PEDIATRIC CLINICS OF NORTH AMERICA Volume 70, Number 5
October 2023 ISSN 0031-3955, ISBN-13: 978-0-323-93903-4

Editor: Kerry Holland
Developmental Editor: Axell Ivan Jade M. Purificacion

Photocopying
Single photocopies of single articles may be made for personal use as allowed by national copyright laws. Permission of the Publisher and payment of a fee is required for all other photocopying, including multiple or systematic copying, copying for advertising or promotional purposes, resale, and all forms of document delivery. Special rates are available for educational institutions that wish to make photocopies for non-profit educational classroom use. For information on how to seek permission visit www.elsevier.com/permissions or call: (+44) 1865 843830 (UK)/(+1) 215 239 3804 (USA).

Derivative Works
Subscribers may reproduce tables of contents or prepare lists of articles including abstracts for internal circulation within their institutions. Permission of the Publisher is required for resale or distribution outside the institution. Permission of the Publisher is required for all other derivative works, including compilations and translations (please consult www.elsevier.com/permissions).

Electronic Storage or Usage
Permission of the Publisher is required to store or use electronically any material contained in this periodical, including any article or part of an article (please consult www.elsevier.com/permissions). Except as outlined above, no part of this publication may be reproduced, stored in a retrieval system or transmitted in any form or by any means, electronic, mechanical, photocopying, recording or otherwise, without prior written permission of the Publisher.

Notice
No responsibility is assumed by the Publisher for any injury and/or damage to persons or property as a matter of products liability, negligence or otherwise, or from any use or operation of any methods, products, instructions or ideas contained in the material herein. Because of rapid advances in the medical sciences, in particular, independent verification of diagnoses and drug dosages should be made.

Although all advertising material is expected to conform to ethical (medical) standards, inclusion in this publication does not constitute a guarantee or endorsement of the quality or value of such product or of the claims made of it by its manufacturer.

The Pediatric Clinics of North America (ISSN 0031-3955) is published bimonthly by Elsevier Inc., 360 Park Avenue South, New York, NY 10010-1710. Months of issue are February, April, June, August, October, and December. Periodicals postage paid at New York, NY and additional mailing offices. Subscription prices are $279.00 per year (US individuals), $827.00 per year (US institutions), $351.00 per year (Canadian individuals), $1100.00 per year (Canadian institutions), $419.00 per year (international individuals), $1100.00 per year (international institutions), $100.00 per year (US students and residents), $100.00 per year (Canadian students and residents), and $165.00 per year (international residents and students). To receive students/resident rate, orders must be accompanied by name of affiliated institution, date of term, and the signature of program/residency coordinator on institution letterhead. Orders will be billed at individual rate until proof of status is received. Foreign air speed delivery is included in all Clinics subscription prices. All prices are subject to change without notice. POSTMASTER: Send address changes to The Pediatric Clinics of North America, Elsevier Health Sciences Division, Subscription Customer Service, 3251 Riverport Lane, Maryland Heights, MO 63043. Customer Service: 1-800-654-2452 (US and Canada). From outside of the US and Canada: 1-314-447-8871. Fax: 1-314-447-8029. For print support, E-mail: JournalsCustomerService-usa@elsevier.com. For online support, E-mail: JournalsOnlineSupport-usa@elsevier.com.

Reprints. For copies of 100 or more, of articles in this publication, please contact the Commercial Reprints Department, Elsevier Inc., 360 Park Avenue South, New York, NY 10010-1710. Tel.: 212-633-3874; Fax: 212-633-3820; E-mail: reprints@elsevier.com.

The Pediatric Clinics of North America is also published in Spanish by McGraw-Hill Inter-americana Editores S.A., Mexico City, Mexico; in Portuguese by Riechmann and Affonso Editores, Rua Comandante Coelho 1085, CEP 21250, Rio de Janeiro, Brazil; and in Greek by Althayia SA, Athens, Greece.

The Pediatric Clinics of North America is covered in MEDLINE/PubMed (Index Medicus), Excerpta Medica, Current Contents, Current Contents/Clinical Medicine, Science Citation Index, ASCA, ISI/BIOMED, and BIOSIS.

PROGRAM OBJECTIVE

The goal of the *Pediatric Clinics of North America* is to keep practicing physicians and residents up to date with current clinical practice in pediatrics by providing timely articles reviewing the state-of-the-art in patient care.

TARGET AUDIENCE

All practicing pediatricians, physicians, and healthcare professionals who provide patient care to pediatric patients.

LEARNING OBJECTIVES

Upon completion of this activity, participants will be able to:

1. Review the substantial benefits of obtaining a genetic diagnosis.
2. Discuss emerging genetic testing and new technologies used to identify challenging variants.
3. Recognize family history and physical exam findings are often the first clues that prompt medical providers to consider clinical genetics evaluation.

ACCREDITATIONS

Physician Credit

The Elsevier Office of Continuing Medical Education (EOCME) is accredited by the Accreditation Council for Continuing Medical Education (ACCME) to provide continuing medical education for physicians.

The EOCME designates this journal-based activity for a maximum of 13 *AMA PRA Category 1 Credit*(s)™. Physicians should claim only the credit commensurate with the extent of their participation in the activity.

All other healthcare professionals requesting continuing education credit for this journal-based activity will be issued a certificate of participation.

ABP Maintenance of Certification Credit

Successful completion of this CME activity, which includes participation in the activity and individual assessment of and feedback to the learner, enables the learner to earn up to 13 MOC points in the American Board of Pediatrics' (ABP) Maintenance of Certification (MOC) program. It is the CME activity provider's responsibility to submit learner completion information to ACCME for the purpose of granting ABP MOC credit.

DISCLOSURE OF CONFLICTS OF INTEREST

The EOCME assesses conflict of interest with its instructors, faculty, planners, and other individuals who are in a position to control the content of CME activities. All relevant conflicts of interest that are identified are thoroughly vetted by EOCME for fair balance, scientific objectivity, and patient care recommendations. EOCME is committed to providing its learners with CME activities that promote improvements or quality in healthcare and not a specific proprietary business or a commercial interest.

The planning committee, staff, authors, and editors listed below have identified no financial relationships or relationships to products or devices they or their spouse/life partner have with commercial interest related to the content of this CME activity:

Peter R. Baker II, MD; Alyce Belonis, MD; Alessandro Blasimme, PhD; Jonathan S. Fletcher, MD, PhD; Arthur L. Lenahan, MD, MPH; Michelle Littlejohn; Pilar L. Magoulas, MS; Rajkumar Mayakrishnan; Kelly E. Ormond, MSc, CGC; Kara Pappas, MD; Natasha Pillay-Smiley, DO; Cynthia A. Prows, MSN, APRN; Nancy Ratner, PhD; Sofia Saenz Ayala, MD; Brian J. Shayota, MD, MPH; Anne Slavotinek, MBBS, PhD; Audrey E. Squire, MS, CGC; Allison Tam, MD; Sonya Tang Girdwood, MD, PhD; Sara Van Driest, MD, PhD; Effy Vayena, PhD

The planning committee, staff, authors, and editors listed below have identified financial relationships or relationships to products or devices they or their spouse/life partner have with commercial interest related to the content of this CME activity:

Andrew Dauber, MD, MMSc: Researcher: BioMarin; Consultant: BioMarin, Pfizer, Inc., Ascendis Pharma, Novo Nordisk

Peter de Blank, MD: Advisor: Alexion Pharmaceuticals, Inc.

Alex Fay, MD,PhD: Consultant: Sarepta, Aeglea, Retrotope, Ultragenyx; Researcher: Sarepta, Elenae; Advisor: Aspiro

Nadia Merchant, MD: Consultant: BioMarin, Pfizer, Inc.

Danny E. Miller, MD, PhD: Researcher, Speaker: Oxford Nanopore Technologies plc; Stock Options: MyOme

Laura B. Ramsey, PhD: Consultant, Researcher: BTG Specialty Pharmaceuticals

UNAPPROVED/OFF-LABEL USE DISCLOSURE
The EOCME requires CME faculty to disclose to the participants:
1. When products or procedures being discussed are off-label, unlabelled, experimental, and/or investigational (not US Food and Drug Administration [FDA] approved); and
2. Any limitations on the information presented, such as data that are preliminary or that represent ongoing research, interim analyses, and/or unsupported opinions. Faculty may discuss information about pharmaceutical agents that is outside of FDA-approved labelling. This information is intended solely for CME and is not intended to promote off-label use of these medications. If you have any questions, contact the medical affairs department of the manufacturer for the most recent prescribing information.

TO ENROLL
To enroll in the *Pediatric Clinics of North America* Continuing Medical Education program, call customer service at 1-800-654-2452 or sign up online at http://www.theclinics.com/home/cme. The CME program is available to subscribers for an additional annual fee of USD 214.00.

METHOD OF PARTICIPATION
In order to claim credit, participants must complete the following:
1. Complete enrolment as indicated above.
2. Read the activity.
3. Complete the CME Test and Evaluation. Participants must achieve a score of 70% on the test. All CME Tests and Evaluations must be completed online.

In order to claim MOC points, participants must complete the following:
1. Complete steps listed above for claiming CME credit
2. Provide your specialty board ID#, birth date (MM/DD), and attestation.
3. Online MOC submission is only available for the American Board of pediatrics' (ABP) Maintenance of Certification (MOC) program

CME INQUIRIES/SPECIAL NEEDS
For all CME inquiries or special needs, please contact elsevierCME@elsevier.com.

Contributors

CONSULTING EDITOR

TINA L. CHENG, MD, MPH
BK Rachford Professor and Chair of Pediatrics, University of Cincinnati, Director, Cincinnati Children's Research Foundation, Chief Medical Officer, Cincinnati Children's Hospital Medical Center, Cincinnati, Ohio, USA

EDITORS

ANNE SLAVOTINEK, MBBS, PhD
Professor of Pediatrics, Medical Genetics, Division of Human Genetics, Cincinnati Children's Hospital Medical Center, Department of Pediatrics, University of Cincinnati School of Medicine, Cincinnati, Ohio, USA

BRITTANY SIMPSON, MD
Assistant Professor, Clinical Geneticist, Division of Human Genetics, Cincinnati Children's Hospital Medical Center, Department of Pediatrics, University of Cincinnati School of Medicine, Cincinnati, Ohio, USA

ALLISON TAM, MD
Assistant Clinical Professor, Division of Medical Genetics, Department of Pediatrics, University of California, San Francisco, San Francisco, California, USA

AUTHORS

PETER R. BAKER II, MD
Associate Professor, Department of Pediatrics, Section of Clinical Genetics and Metabolism, University of Colorado, Children's Hospital Colorado, Aurora, Colorado, USA

ALYCE BELONIS, MD
Assistant Professor, Division of Human Genetics, Cincinnati Children's Hospital Medical Center, Department of Pediatrics, University of Cincinnati School of Medicine, Cincinnati, Ohio, USA

ALESSANDRO BLASIMME, PhD
Senior Scientist, Department of Health Sciences and Technology, Health Ethics and Policy Lab, ETH Zurich, Zurich, Switzerland

ANDREW DAUBER, MD, MMSc
Division of Endocrinology, Children's National Hospital, Department of Pediatrics, George Washington University School of Medicine and Health Sciences, Washington, DC, USA

PETER DE BLANK, MD
Professor of Pediatrics, Cancer and Blood Diseases Institute, The Cure Starts Now Foundation Brain Tumor Center, Division of Experimental Hematology and Cancer Biology, Cancer and Blood Diseases Institute, Cincinnati Children's Hospital Medical Center, University of Cincinnati College of Medicine, Cincinnati, Ohio, USA

ALEX FAY, MD, PhD
Associate Professor of Neurology, University of California, San Francisco, San Francisco, California, USA

JONATHAN S. FLETCHER, MD, PhD
Division of Experimental Hematology and Cancer Biology, Cancer and Blood Diseases Institute, Cincinnati Children's Hospital Medical Center, University of Cincinnati College of Medicine, Cincinnati, Ohio, USA; Division of Hematology-Oncology, University of Texas Southwestern, Dallas, Texas USA

ARTHUR L. LENAHAN, MD, MPH
Division of Genetic Medicine, Department of Pediatrics, University of Washington, Seattle Children's Hospital, Seattle, Washington, USA

PILAR L. MAGOULAS, MS, CGC
Associate Professor, Chief, Division of Genetic Counseling, Department of Molecular and Human Genetics, Baylor College of Medicine, Texas Children's Hospital, Houston, Texas, USA

NADIA MERCHANT, MD
Division of Endocrinology, Children's National Hospital, Department of Pediatrics, George Washington University School of Medicine and Health Sciences, Washington, DC, USA

DANNY E. MILLER, MD, PhD
Division of Genetic Medicine, Department of Pediatrics, Seattle Children's Hospital, Department of Laboratory Medicine and Pathology, University of Washington, Seattle, Washington, USA

KELLY E. ORMOND, MS, CGC
Research Scientist and ABGC/EBMG Credentialed Genetic Counselor, Department of Health Sciences and Technology, Health Ethics and Policy Lab, ETH Zurich, Zurich, Switzerland; Adjunct Professor, Department of Genetics, Stanford Center for Biomedical Ethics, Stanford University School of Medicine, Stanford, California, USA

KARA B. PAPPAS, MD
Division of Genetics, Genomics and Metabolic Disorders, Children's Hospital of Michigan, Detroit, Michigan, USA; Assistant Professor, Department of Pediatrics, Central Michigan University, Mount Pleasant, Michigan, USA

NATASHA PILLAY-SMILEY, DO
Assistant Professor of Pediatrics, Cancer and Blood Diseases Institute, The Cure Starts Now Foundation Brain Tumor Center, Division of Experimental Hematology and Cancer Biology, Cincinnati Children's Hospital Medical Center, University of Cincinnati College of Medicine, Cincinnati, Ohio, USA

CYNTHIA A. PROWS, MSN, APRN
Clinical Nurse Specialist, Division of Human Genetics, Department of Pediatrics, Center for Professional Excellence, Patient Services, Cincinnati Children's Hospital Medical Center, College of Medicine, University of Cincinnati, Cincinnati, Ohio, USA

LAURA B. RAMSEY, PhD
Associate Professor, Divisions of Clinical Pharmacology, and Research in Patient Services, Cincinnati Children's Hospital Medical Center, Department of Pediatrics, University of Cincinnati College of Medicine, Cincinnati, Ohio, USA

NANCY RATNER, PhD
Professor of Pediatrics, Division of Experimental Hematology and Cancer Biology, Cancer and Blood Diseases Institute, Cincinnati Children's Hospital Medical Center, University of Cincinnati College of Medicine, Cincinnati, Ohio, USA

SOFIA SAENZ AYALA, MD
Assistant Professor, Division of Human Genetics, University of Maryland Medical Center, Baltimore, Maryland, USA

BRIAN J. SHAYOTA, MD, MPH
Assistant Professor, University of Utah, Primary Children's Hospital, Salt Lake City, Utah, USA

ANNE SLAVOTINEK, MBBS, PhD
Professor of Pediatrics, Medical Genetics, Division of Human Genetics, Cincinnati Children's Hospital Medical Center, Department of Pediatrics, University of Cincinnati School of Medicine, Cincinnati, Ohio

AUDREY E. SQUIRE, MS, CGC
Division of Genetic Medicine, Department of Pediatrics, University of Washington, Seattle Children's Hospital, Seattle, Washington, USA

ALLISON TAM, MD
Assistant Clinical Professor, Division of Medical Genetics, Department of Pediatrics, University of California, San Francisco, San Francisco, California, USA

SONYA TANG GIRDWOOD, MD, PhD
Assistant Professor, Divisions of Hospital Medicine, and Clinical Pharmacology, Cincinnati Children's Hospital Medical Center, Department of Pediatrics, University of Cincinnati College of Medicine, Cincinnati, Ohio, USA

SARA VAN DRIEST, MD, PhD
Associate Professor of Pediatrics and Medicine, Department of Pediatrics, Vanderbilt University Medical Center, Nashville, Tennessee, USA

EFFY VAYENA, PhD
Professor and Deputy Head of Institute of Translational Medicine, Department of Health Sciences and Technology, Health Ethics and Policy Lab, ETH Zurich, Zurich, Switzerland

Contents

> In the last few decades, medical genetics has undergone a revolution because of the development of technologies and informatics approaches that can generate and analyze large amounts of genomic data. Pediatricians have been hugely affected by these changes. The early age of presentation for birth defects and neurocognitive disorders, together with a shortage of trained genetics professionals, has increased consultations for conditions with a genetic cause, not only in pediatric practice but also in other subspecialties. In the future, genetic testing in childhood is likely to include pediatricians, who can initiate testing in partnership with trained genetics professionals.

> Although genetics has traditionally been associated with pregnancy, birth defects, and newborn screening, almost every disease is influenced in part by an individual's genetic makeup. Therefore, it is important to consider the impact of genetics in health and disease throughout an individual's lifetime.

> Selecting the ideal test to evaluate an individual with a suspected genetic disorder can be challenging. While several clinical testing options are available, no single test yet captures all potentially causative genetic variants. Thus, clinicians may order testing in a stepwise fashion, and what to order after non-diagnostic testing can be challenging to determine. Here, we provide an overview of commonly used clinical genetic tests, guidance on when they are best used, and what they may miss. We conclude with a discussion of how new technologies might be used to identify challenging variants and simplify clinical testing in the future.

Receiving a genetic diagnosis can be challenging for parents as they learn to cope and adapt to this news. They often experience a myriad of emotions ranging from shock to relief. Yet overwhelmingly, parents report a negative experience with this process. Factors that improve parental satisfaction include being provided written information, emotional and psychosocial support, and connections with other parents. Genetics care providers are particularly equipped to solicit parental needs and provide support before, during, and after receiving a diagnosis. This review will provide suggestions and recommendations for supporting parents throughout the diagnostic testing experience and receiving a genetic diagnosis.

As the availability of advanced molecular testing like whole exome and genome sequencing expands, it comes with the added complication of interpreting inconclusive results, including determining the relevance of variants of uncertain significance or failing to find a variant in an otherwise suspected specific genetic disorder. This complication necessitates the use of alternative testing methods to gather more information in support of, or against, a particular genetic diagnosis. Therefore, new genome-wide approaches, including DNA epigenetic testing, RNA sequencing, and metabolomics, are increasingly being used to increase the diagnostic yield when used in conjunction with more conventional genetic tests.

Neurofibromatosis type I (NF1) is a common dominantly inherited disorder, and one of the most common of the RASopathies. Most individuals with NF1 develop plexiform neurofibromas and cutaneous neurofibromas, nerve tumors caused by NF1 loss of function in Schwann cells. Cell culture models and mouse models of NF1 are being used to test drug efficacy in preclinical trials, which led to Food and Drug Administration approval for use of Selumetinib (a MEK inhibitor) to shrink most inoperable plexiform neurofibromas. This article details methods used for testing in preclinical models, and outlines newer models that may identify additional, curative, strategies.

Achondroplasia is the most common form of disproportionate severe short stature. Management of achondroplasia requires a multidisciplinary approach and has been largely symptomatic for medical complications and psychosocial implications. Increased understanding of genetic and molecular mechanisms of achondroplasia has led to the development of novel disease-modifying drugs. The current drugs under investigation target the growth plate to stimulate chondrocyte growth and development. These include analogs of C-type natriuretic peptide (CNP), FGFR3-selective tyrosine kinase inhibitors, anti-FGFR3 antibodies, aptamers against FGF2, and soluble forms of FGFR3. Long-term data on the effects of these therapies on medical comorbidities are pending at this time.

Spinal muscular atrophy (SMA) is a progressive disease of the lower motor neurons associated with recessive loss of the *SMN1* gene, and which leads to worsening weakness and disability, and is fatal in its most severe forms. Over the past six years, three treatments have emerged, two drugs that modify exon splicing and one gene therapy, which have transformed the management of this disease. When treated pre-symptomatically, many children show normal early motor development, and the benefits extend from the newborn period to adulthood. Similar treatment approaches are now under investigation for rare types of SMA associated with genes beyond *SMN1*.

In some relatively common inborn errors of metabolism there can be the accumulation of toxic compounds including ammonia and organic acids such as lactate and ketoacids, as well as energy deficits at the cellular level. The clinical presentation is often referred to as a metabolic emergency or crisis. Fasting and illness can result in encephalopathy within hours, and without appropriate recognition and intervention, the outcome may be permanent disability or death. This review outlines easy and readily available means of recognizing and diagnosing a metabolic emergency as well as general guidelines for management. Disease-specific interventions focus on parenteral nutrition to reverse catabolism, toxin removal strategies, and vitamin/nutrition supplementation.

Pharmacogenomics, where genomic information is used to tailor medication management, is a strategy to maximize drug efficacy and minimize toxicity. Although pediatric evidence is less robust than for adults, medications influenced by pharmacogenomics are prescribed to children and adolescents. Evidence-based guidelines and drug label annotations are available from the Clinical Pharmacogenetics Implementation Consortium (CPIC) and the Pharmacogenomics Knowledgebase (PharmGKB). Some pediatric health care facilities use pharmacogenomics to provide dosing recommendations to pediatricians. Herein, we use a case-based approach to illustrate the use of pharmacogenomic data in pediatric clinical care and provide resources for finding and using pharmacogenomic guidelines.

The goal of newborn screening is to identify medical conditions that can cause significant morbidity and/or mortality if not treated early in life. Pediatricians often play a vital role in the initial disclosure of newborn screening results and coordination of confirmatory testing, treatment, and referral to specialty care. The goal of this article is to provide an overview of current newborn screening in the United States, focusing on the various disorders, their manifestations, the newborn screening process, the confirmatory testing, and treatments. Some practical considerations will be discussed as well.

Pediatric health care providers caring for patients and families with genetic disease will encounter a range of ethical issues. These include traditional pediatric health care issues, such as surrogate decision making and end-of-life care. Genetic testing raises the importance of informed consent for potential risks that move beyond the oft discussed physical risks and into longer term concepts such as psychological impact, privacy and potential discrimination. Predictive testing in childhood also raises questions of whether the child has an autonomy interest in delaying testing until they have decision making capacity to do so on their own. And finally, treatments including gene therapies and gene editing, may raise issues of identity for families dealing with genetic disease.

Family history and physical exam findings are often the first clues that prompt medical providers to consider clinical genetics evaluation. There is standardized nomenclature for both the pedigree and description of physical features. Systematic evaluation of patients through obtaining family history and careful physical examination is essential to the formulation of a differential diagnosis and plan in the clinical genetics evaluation. The goal of this article is to provide an overview of family history and dysmorphology exam, and their relevance for the clinical genetics evaluation.

PEDIATRIC CLINICS OF NORTH AMERICA

THE CLINICS ARE AVAILABLE ONLINE!
Access your subscription at:
www.theclinics.com

Foreword

The Promise of the Genomics Revolution in Pediatrics

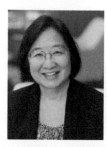

Tina L. Cheng, MD, MPH
Consulting Editor

With the sequencing of the human genome in 2003, we are now realizing the promise of genetic medicine. Previous NIH Director Elias Zerhouni suggested that with genetic molecular preemption we are experiencing a paradigm shift for medicine characterized by "4 P's": predictive, preemptive, participatory, and personalized care, and a shifting of focus earlier in the life course.[1,2] I have previously written that the fifth "P" is Pediatrics, as this is the life stage where molecular preemption has the best potential to influence health risk,[3] and a sixth "P" is Prenatal. Prenatal and pediatric care are at the leading edge of the promise of the genomics revolution combined with knowledge of other psychosocial and environmental influences on health. As clinicians, we must embrace the opportunity to implement the 6 "P's" to predict the emergence of future health conditions and prevent, preempt, and buffer negative outcomes while optimizing a positive health trajectory.

It seems like almost every pediatric journal issue these days reports new genes with phenotype-causing mutations and discovery of phenotypes with known molecular basis. Genome sequencing has become standard of care in a growing number of medical conditions and with high diagnostic yield in many conditions, including pediatric rare diseases.[4] Keeping up with this explosion of information to serve our patients and

Pediatr Clin N Am 70 (2023) xv–xvi
https://doi.org/10.1016/j.pcl.2023.07.001
0031-3955/23/© 2023 Published by Elsevier Inc.

families can be a challenge. This issue can help in discussing the current status and the ethical and equity issues to also consider.

Tina L. Cheng, MD, MPH
University of Cincinnati
Cincinnati Children's Research Foundation
Cincinnati Children's Hospital
Medical Center
3333 Burnet Avenue, MLC 3016
Cincinnati, OH 45229-3026, USA

E-mail address:
Tina.cheng@cchmc.org

REFERENCES

1. Zerhouni E. A vision for transforming medicine in the 21st century. Available at: http://www.nih.gov/about/director/slides/vision.pdf. Accessed October 12, 2007.
2. Zerhouni E. Breakfast with Dr. Zerhouni video. Available at: https://www.google.com/search?q=elias+zerhouni+4+p&rlz=1C1GCEB_enUS931US931&oq=elias+zerhouni+4+p&gs_lcrp=EgZjaHJvbWUyBggAEEUYOTIGCAEQRRhA0gEINTgyN2oxajSoAgCwAgA&sourceid=chrome&ie=UTF-8#fpstate=ive&vld=cid:e8aa8453,vid:-b3VlozaAc8. Accessed May 14, 2023.
3. Cheng TL, Cohn RD, Dover GJ. The genetics revolution and primary care pediatrics: the 6 P's. JAMA 2008;299(4):451-3.
4. Wright CF, Campbell P, Eberhardt RY, et al, DDD Study. Genomic diagnosis of rare pediatric disease in the United Kingdom and Ireland. N Engl J Med 2023;388(17):1559-71. https://doi.org/10.1056/NEJMoa2209046.

Preface

Genetics in Pediatric Practice

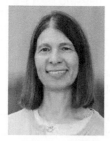
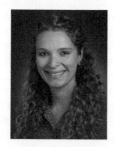
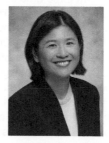

Anne Slavotinek, MBBS, PhD   Brittany Simpson, MD   Allison Tam, MD
Editors

In this issue of *Pediatric Clinics of North America*, we celebrate the importance of Genetics in Pediatric Practice and provide information for pediatricians who are at the forefront of managing the care of patients with genetic disorders. The issue starts with the article by Dr Anne Slavotinek, "Genetics in Pediatric Practice, from Baby Steps to Running Fast." This work discusses the future of precision medicine in pediatric care and the consideration that pediatricians may play a more active role in initiating genetic testing in the future. The article "Genetics 101—When to Refer," by Drs Alyce Belonis and Sofia Saenz Ayala, provides a refresher on the indications for referrals to genetics professionals in light of an evolving and increasing range of genetic testing options and treatments. Referral indications, including physical anomalies, birth defects, abnormal growth patterns, reproductive history, developmental delays and autism, inborn errors of metabolism, and medical history suggestive of a predisposition to cancer or a prior genetic diagnosis, are discussed. The next few articles reflect topics that might arise as a patient and family navigate findings suggestive of a genetic condition and the start of the diagnostic odyssey. "Panels, Exomes, Genomes, and More—Finding the Best Path Through the Diagnostic Odyssey," by Dr Arthur L. Lenahan, Ms Audrey E. Squire, and Dr Danny E. Miller, summarizes current genetic testing technologies and factors influencing test selection for pediatric and genetic health professionals. The article examines the mainstay of genetic investigations with chromosomal approaches, gene panel testing, and exome and genome sequencing, together with testing for imprinting disorders and repeat expansions. The article concludes with a brief introduction to newer technologies, including optical genome mapping and long-read genome sequencing. In the article entitled "Supporting Families Through the Genetic Testing Process and New Diagnosis," by Ms Pilar L. Magoulas, a framework for how best to support patients and families through the experience of obtaining a new genetic diagnosis is developed. The material includes tips for breaking challenging news and for the psychosocial support of families adapting and adjusting to a new diagnosis. The

Pediatr Clin N Am 70 (2023) xvii–xix
https://doi.org/10.1016/j.pcl.2023.06.004
0031-3955/23/© 2023 Published by Elsevier Inc.

article by Dr Brian J. Shayota, "Downstream Assays for Variant Resolution: Epigenetics, RNA Sequencing, and Metabolomics," introduces the principles underlying ancillary testing for variant resolution after inconclusive genetic testing results. This article describes postexome strategies involving epigenetics, transcriptomics with RNA-seq, and metabolomics.

The subsequent three articles, grouped under the heading, "Shedding New Light—Novel Therapies for Common Disorders," discuss gene- and pathway-specific treatments for commonly encountered disorders in pediatric practice. The article written by Dr Natasha Pillay-Smiley, Dr Jonathan S. Fletcher, Dr Peter de Blank, and Dr Nancy Ratner discusses "Neurofibromatosis Type I" (NF1), including common clinical findings, predisposition to malignancy, relationship to other rasopathies, and animal models of the disease. The article then summarizes the research and clinical use of newer treatments, such as MEK inhibitors for NF1 and other rasopathies. The article written by Drs Andrew Dauber and Nadia Merchant examines "Achondroplasia and Growth Disorders," with a description of clinical features of achondroplasia and FGFR3-related disorders, management guidelines, and therapy with growth hormone and C-natriuretic peptide (CNP) analogues comprising vosoritide and TransCon-CNP. The article also discusses infigratinib, an FGFR1-3 inhibitor, and recifercept, an FGFR3 decoy, along with other emerging therapies. Dr Alexander Fay explores "Spinal Muscular Atrophy," including a history of the disorder, a description of the clinical features, and different types of spinal muscular atrophy, the genetic cause of the condition, clinical trials, and targeted therapies with nusinersen, onasemnogene abeparvovec, and risdiplam.

The next group of articles covers clinical situations involving genetic disorders, ranging from metabolic crises to newborn screening and pharmacogenomics. In "Recognizing and Managing a Metabolic Crisis," written by Dr. Peter Barker II, current strategies for the acute management of patients with the most frequent inborn errors of metabolism are covered, here comprising urea cycle disorders, organic acidemias, maple syrup urine disease, fatty acid oxidation disorders, and primary lactic acidosis. In "Current Practices in Pharmacogenomics," written by Dr Laura B. Ramsey, Ms Cynthia A. Prows, Dr Sonya Tang Girdwood, and Dr Sara Van Driest, guidelines available for using pharmacogenomics to manage medications in pediatric patients are summarized. This article provides examples of contemporary dilemmas in pediatric pharmacogenomics practice, including complex patients and patients with neurologic disorders, children undergoing surgery or receiving oncologic treatments, and those with rare genetic diseases. Dr Kara Pappas reports updates in "Newborn Screening" that are critical for identifying early-onset disorders with effective treatments. This article discusses screening for hearing loss, critical congenital heart disease, hemoglobinopathies, cystic fibrosis, endocrinologic conditions (hypothyroidism and congenital adrenal hyperplasia), immunologic conditions (severe combined immunodeficiency), and inborn errors of metabolism.

In "Ethical Aspects of Pediatric Genetic Care: Testing and Treatment," by Ms Kelly E. Ormond, Dr Effy Vayena, and Dr Alessandro Blasimme, definitions of ethical principles and common ethical considerations in Pediatric practice, such as informed consent, autonomy, and unsolicited findings, are provided. The article also mentions clinical examples and discusses ethical situations in the newborn period and at the end of life, with mention of data-sharing and privacy in addition to other ethical questions that can arise during genetic testing and results disclosure. Last, the compilation ends with an overview of some of the basic skills required for successful implementation of genetics into pediatric practice. "Essential Pieces to the Genetics Puzzle:

Family History and Dysmorphology Exam," by Dr Allison Tam, looks at the importance of taking an accurate family history and correctly describing physical anomalies.

Medical genetics today is an information and technology–rich specialty that can provide molecular genetic diagnoses and treatments for an ever-increasing range of disorders. Pediatricians will continue to be on the front line of this revolution, in terms of ascertaining patients with genetic conditions and managing their care. The shortage of medical genetics professionals makes it desirable that pediatricians become familiar with genetic practices. We hope you enjoy this work and provide our heartfelt thanks to all of the authors and reviewers for their contributions.

Anne Slavotinek, MBBS, PhD
Division of Human Genetics
Cincinnati Children's Hospital Medical Center
Department of Pediatrics
University of Cincinnati School of Medicine
3333 Burnet Avenue, ML4006
Cincinnati, OH 45229, USA

Brittany Simpson, MD
Division of Human Genetics
Cincinnati Children's Hospital Medical Center
Department of Pediatrics
University of Cincinnati School of Medicine
3333 Burnet Avenue, ML4006
Cincinnati, OH 45229, USA

Allison Tam, MD
Division of Medical Genetics
Department of Pediatrics
University of California, San Francisco
UCSF Benioff Children's Hospital
550 16th Street, 4th Floor
San Francisco, CA 94143, USA

E-mail addresses:
anne.slavotinek@cchmc.org (A. Slavotinek)
brittany.simpson@cchmc.org (B. Simpson)
Allison.tam@ucsf.edu (A. Tam)

Genetics in Pediatric Practice

From Baby Steps to Running Fast

Anne Slavotinek, MBBS, PhD

KEYWORDS

- Exome sequencing • Rapid genome sequencing • Secondary and incidental findings
- Genetics education

KEY POINTS

- Pediatricians need to be vigilant to recognize clinical situations that warrant genetic testing or a genetics referral.
- Care models are changing for genetic disorders, and it is likely that pediatricians will increasingly be involved in ordering and interpreting genetic tests in the future.
- Future educational opportunities for pediatricians are likely to be collaborative and take advantage of newer technologies, such as telehealth.

INTRODUCTION

In 2022, the 200th anniversary of Gregor Mendel's birthday, rare diseases with Mendelian inheritance patterns could not be more important in pediatric care. The initial draft map of the human genome was completed in 2001,[1,2] and the first "full sequence" was published in 2003 to usher in a new era of genomic medicine.[3] The most complete reference assembly of the human genome has only recently been published and is an important step toward models of the genome that represent diverse ancestries.[4] These reference sequences for the human genome have formed part of a molecular toolbox that has been immensely helpful for the interpretation of genetic data.[5] At the same time, next-generation array and sequencing methodologies that produce abundant genomic data have developed in parallel, including arrays for genome-wide association studies, microarrays for detecting copy number variants,[6] exome sequencing (ES),[7] and genome sequencing (GS).[8] Medical genetics has therefore become less focused on recognizing clinical patterns and diseases and instead more concentrated on obtaining and analyzing genetic data. As costs of testing

Medical Genetics, Division of Human Genetics, Department of Pediatrics, Cincinnati Children's Hospital Medical Center, University of Cincinnati School of Medicine, 3333 Burnet Avenue, Cincinnati, OH 45229, USA
E-mail address: anne.slavotinek@cchmc.org

Pediatr Clin N Am 70 (2023) 885–894
https://doi.org/10.1016/j.pcl.2023.05.003
pediatric.theclinics.com

continue to decrease, genetic testing has become more accessible and the ability to compile data from unrelated patients with rare Mendelian disorders has accelerated the discovery of numerous human disease genes.[9] In recent years, the field has further expanded from a discipline largely focused on single-gene disorders to encompass more common, multifactorial diseases that are influenced by multiple genetic susceptibility factors.[10] Genetic diseases and the contribution of genetic factors to complex conditions are now relevant to almost all medical subspecialties and health care practitioners.

Precision medicine can be defined as an emerging practice of medicine that uses an individual's genetic profile (and artificial intelligence) to guide decisions made in regard to the prevention, diagnosis, and treatment of disease.[11] Because pediatricians are involved in the management and treatment of patients with rare disorders, they are ideally situated to use precision medicine and translate genetic information into changes in care. Many rare disorders are first detected in the neonatal period or early childhood, and the multitude of new syndromes in this population has greatly influenced pediatric practice. The early age of onset of many genetic conditions necessitates the involvement of pediatricians and other specialists in the process of genetic referral and diagnosis. This review focuses on the importance of genetic testing in pediatric practice and the suggestion that pediatricians should play an active role in initiating these investigations. Strategies for educating pediatricians and other subspecialty providers in genetics and genomics are also discussed. A detailed description of the methodologies for genetic testing is provided in Arthur L. Lenahan and colleagues' article, "Panels, Exomes, Genomes and more—Finding the Best Path Through the Diagnostic Odyssey," in this issue; other considerations relating to genetic testing that are covered in this collection include an article on when to refer to genetics (see Alyce Belonis and Sofia Saenz Ayala's article, "Genetics 101: When to Refer," in this issue), practices for supporting families through the genetic testing odyssey (see Pilar L. Magoulas' article, "Supporting Parents Throughout the Genetic Testing Process and New Diagnosis," in this issue), and tips for obtaining a family history and dysmorphology assessment (see Allison Tam's article, "Essential Pieces to the Genetics Puzzle: Family History and Dysmorphology Exam," in this issue).

GENETIC TESTING: MORE COMPREHENSIVE AND MORE RAPID

Pediatricians are the primary care providers for patients presenting with medical illnesses or for surveillance during the formative years from birth throughout childhood to early adult life. Pediatricians have long needed to be familiar with many aspects of genetics, because they, together with other primary care providers, are often the first to be consulted regarding genetic conditions affecting children or families.[12] Genetic testing, including microarrays, gene panels, ES, and GS, is becoming increasingly used in younger age groups because of improved insurance coverage,[13] a high diagnostic yield, and actionability of genetic testing results early in life.[14]

The advent of next-generation sequencing technologies and the trend toward offering broad genetic testing as a rapid test is highly relevant to pediatric care during the neonatal period. Infants admitted for intensive care after birth can be critically ill, with nonspecific clinical presentations, such as encephalopathy or recurrent seizures. The phenotypic findings at presentation may also not resemble those of the final underlying diagnosis.[15] A broad testing strategy that covers both copy number variants and single nucleotide variants is therefore justified. Rapid ES and GS are now frequently sent from the neonatal intensive care unit (NICU) or nursery, and these tests have become increasingly popular because of their power to cover numerous conditions and provide a fast diagnosis.[15–19] In addition, the impressive diagnostic rates of ES and GS suggest a high prevalence of genetic disease in the NICU that is likely to be underestimated.[16] Diagnostic rates can be as high as 40% for infants receiving rapid GS and accomplished in as little as 3 days.[20] Studies of varying size and on babies in different health care systems have shown that a molecular genetic diagnosis changes management and alters medical decision making in as many as 83% of infants.[15,19] The benefits of receiving a positive result are well described, and several are listed in the following discussion.

Benefits of Identifying a Causative Genetic Variant

- Treatment directed at the underlying genetic cause
- Disease-specific surveillance
- Provision of support services
- Family planning and reproductive counseling
- Access to clinical trials and natural history studies
- Research participation

A negative result may also be helpful, because almost all currently known disease-causing genes can be ruled out,[15] although a negative result may do little to allay the suspicion of an underlying genetic condition held by an experienced clinician. It has been thought that the greatest potential contribution of GS to human health is from testing undertaken in the newborn period, but the optimal breadth of genetic testing in NICUs of different levels remains undetermined.[16]

CHALLENGES FOR IMPLEMENTING GENETIC TESTING

Despite the advantages of rapid, comprehensive testing, there remain diagnostic limitations to rapid ES and GS testing. Ancillary testing is still sometimes needed, because next-generation sequencing tests can still fail to detect relatively common conditions with a genetic cause, such as the homozygous exon 7 and 8 deletions in SMN1 that cause spinal muscular atrophy type 1, methylation defects associated with Beckwith-Wiedemann syndrome, and low-level mosaicism.[15] Although obtaining truly informed consent in acute care settings is problematic,[21] this difficulty is not unique to genetic testing and concerns about breaches in confidentiality and later discrimination[22] are still largely unrealized. Caring for children who have been diagnosed with rare diseases without clear clinical management guidelines can be challenging (**Table 1**), but this situation is no different from the pediatric practice and

Table 1	
Challenges caring for children with genetic conditions	
Challenges	**Possible Approaches**
• Difficulty in obtaining specialist care	• Access to genetics providers through telemedicine
• Lack of insurance coverage for genetic testing	• Free testing programs through sponsoring companies
• Time lag for testing results/ segregation testing in parents	• Sending parental samples with patient samples
• Risk of test/variant misinterpretation	• Information from testing laboratories; specialist consultations
• Paucity of information about rare conditions	• Contact advocacy groups and researchers
• Lack of support groups and resources for different population groups	• Online rare disease networks such as National Organization for Rare Disorders

care that has occurred throughout the ages. Having a diagnosis is the first critical step in designing treatments, and the practical benefits arising from diagnostic genetic information can be substantial, as listed earlier.[16] The sheer power of ES and GS to obtain an answer in critical diagnostic situations means that these tests will continue to be an increasingly used and a vital component of pediatric care.

The important role of the pediatrician in detecting early growth delays, developmental differences, and behavioral challenges that can constitute the clinical signs of an underlying genetic disorder remains unchanged. Many pediatricians are skilled at identifying the patterns of physical anomalies and differences from typical neurodevelopmental trajectories that constitute the features of a genetic syndrome. The role for early recognition and accurate phenotyping is as crucial as ever for identifying situations in which genetic testing should be considered. In addition, careful posttest phenotyping focusing on diagnoses suggested by the genetic testing results remains essential for accurate test interpretation, even for pathogenic and likely pathogenic variants, for which a diagnosis is frequently assumed regardless of the phenotype.[23]

INITIATING GENETIC TESTING IS NOT JUST FOR GENETICS PROFESSIONALS

The shortage of genetic specialists in the United States[24–26] and long waiting times for specialist care suggests that nongenetics providers, such as pediatricians and primary care providers, now need to feel comfortable ordering genetic testing. The author envisages that pediatricians alongside other health care providers are likely to play a major role in initiating genetic testing and reducing the diagnostic odyssey in the future. Genomic testing in the NICU has been met with a high degree of satisfaction from providers and patients alike.[16] If a genomic test ordered by a pediatrician results in a clear diagnosis, with a pathogenic or likely pathogenic variant that explains the clinical presentation, referral to a genetics service or specialist disease center can be undertaken without delay. The genetics service or specialist center can then provide care relevant to the genetic diagnosis, such as starting or stopping treatments, providing management advice, answering parent and family questions, facilitating participation in natural history studies, and providing connections with researchers and support groups. If the genomic test does not result in a diagnosis and either returns a variant of uncertain significance (VUS) or a negative result, then referral to a genetics service may still be appropriate, because the genetics professional can evaluate the remaining likelihood of a genetic disorder and ensure that the genomic testing already sent was appropriate. Because genetic testing frequently takes weeks or months to return results, referral to a genetic service as early as the time of test ordering will facilitate timely follow-up. The traditionally slow processes of a genetics referral and genomic testing are thus expedited. This time saved can be a critical factor for infants and young children, in whom several months of lost time could equate to a considerable proportion of their elapsed life span. One hurdle to implementing genetic testing is ensuring that there is insurance coverage, although with decreasing costs and increasing use it is fair to hope that this barrier will diminish with time. A simple strategy of short and directed, combined telehealth visits by a pediatrician and a genetics specialist may facilitate the documentation needed for insurance approval and have the advantage of introducing a future specialist to the family.

An approach that delegates the initiation of genetic testing to the sphere of pediatrics and primary care is still controversial. Despite high diagnostic utility and a direct effect on clinical management for 90.6% (29 of 32) of patients in one study, the investigators still recommended an initial genetics consultation in the NICU before testing owing to the high costs associated with genetic investigations and the possibility of alternative diagnostic strategies.[27] Others have been more forthright about the benefits that can accrue from prompt genetic testing in terms of high diagnostic and clinical utility and cost-effectiveness, maintaining that a high index of suspicion for genetic disorders should be upheld for any unexplained symptoms.[28] Support from genetics professionals is also highly relevant for any genetic testing performed by outside providers.[28]

PEDIATRICIANS AND GENETICISTS: LEARNING ON THE JOB

For health professionals who are not primarily trained in genetics, the practice of providing a gateway to precision medicine can be daunting. Complicated and nuanced results, such as VUSs, secondary findings, incidental findings, and variants in novel disease genes, often require a sophisticated understanding of genetic concepts and can be demanding even for trained genetics providers.[14] There can be a clear need for pediatricians to partner with those experienced in genetic conditions so that the downstream care for families affected by genetic diseases is shared. However, it is not typical for pediatricians to have undergone formal training in medical genetics. Many nongenetics providers may feel unprepared to help their patients decide whether genetic testing is needed, which tests to order, how to interpret the results, and how to apply the said results to improve patient care and outcomes.[29] Only one-third of respondents in one study agreed that their training prepared them to work with genetically high-risk patients, and even fewer (15%) felt confident in their ability to use genetic results in practice.[30] Numerous studies have reported that nongeneticist physicians perceive that they lack the knowledge and skillsets to implement genomic medicine in their practices and less than one-quarter (23%) of physician respondents agreed they could find and use reliable sources of information to understand and communicate genetic risk in the care of their patients.[30] Nisselle and colleagues[31] surveyed 409 Australian medical specialists that represented 30 specialties, 20% of whom were pediatricians. Although more than half of the specialists (53.9%) had engaged in genetic testing over the preceding 12 months, either by ordering a test or referring a patient for genetic services, survey respondents lacked confidence in their knowledge and ability to explain genomic concepts and to make decisions based on genomic information.[31] In contrast, the specialists described the highest level of confidence in taking a family history to elicit information about genetic conditions.[31]

Even if partnering with a geneticist, how should pediatricians and other nongeneticist health care providers go forward if they have an interest in learning more about genetics?

Strategies for Nongenetics Professionals to Familiarize Themselves with Genetics

- Self-education, including reading of specialty text and articles
- Educational materials and programs from specialist societies
- Seminars and departmental presentations
- Clinical meetings and conferences
- Shared care and learning from peers
- Specific educational workshops

There are many resources for self-education about individual genetic conditions (**Table 2**), as well as information on basic genetic terminology, genetic report interpretation,[14] and pedigree drawing.[32] Specialized programs, such as those funded by the Association of Public Health Laboratories' Newborn Screening Technical

Table 2
Educational resources for pediatric consultations for genetic disorders in childhood

	Examples of Educational Resources
Neonatal period • Positive newborn screening results • Down syndrome • Birth defects • Metabolic conditions	• Newborn screening: ACTion (ACT) sheets and algorithms, Newborn Screening Translational Research Network • Down syndrome: National Down Syndrome Society • Birth defects resources: National Institute of Child Health and Development • Metabolic conditions: Society for Inherited Metabolic Disease
Early childhood • Developmental delays • Growth delays • Autism and behavioral differences • Seizure disorders • Hearing loss	• Genetic conditions: Medline • Variant interpretation guidelines[46] • Autism: Simons Foundation • Hearing loss: American Speech-Language-Hearing Association • Seizure disorders: National Association of Epilepsy Centers
Late childhood/adolescence • Turner syndrome • Klinefelter syndrome • Mitochondrial conditions	• Turner syndrome and Klinefelter syndrome: Pediatric Endocrine Society • Mitochondrial conditions: United Mitochondrial Disease Foundation

Assistance and Evaluation Program (NewSTEPs)[33] and the American College of Medical Genetics and Genomics ACTion (ACT) Sheets that are supported by the National Coordinating Center for the Regional Genetics Networks, also provide educational material for pediatricians. However, these information sources require interpretation and may not help providers without access to resources for questions. In their survey of Australian medical specialists, Nisselle and colleagues[31] found that preferred modes of learning about genomics included incorporating genetics education into work activities in the form of seminars, departmental presentations, and clinical meetings, together with learning from peers. Continuing professional development was also favored, but reading specialty texts, although frequent, was rated as less helpful.[31] Distance learning courses in genetics and genomics practice have also been successful and can result in improved knowledge in the immediate and midterm time scale up to 8 months.[34] Interactive workshops and educational modules also improve the knowledge and confidence needed to deliver genetic services in primary care settings.[35] Evaluation of an interactive Web-based curriculum focusing on risk assessment and genetic testing; ethical, legal, and social implications (ELSI); and communication and practice behaviors resulted in improved decision making and increased ELSI discussions with patients.[36] However, brief educational interventions may not impact clinician behaviors in the long term.[37] After an initial assessment by a pediatrician, shared care models with collaborative telemedicine encounters between pediatricians and geneticists may also provide opportunities for learning and help to overcome the shortage of genetics providers.[38] Many practitioners would like contact with genetic professionals to answer questions,[35] and genetics professionals should also be included alongside pediatricians and other care providers in patient-centered medical homes to help coordinate the management of complex or chronic genetic conditions.[38] A negative correlation between time from acquiring a medical degree and knowledge of "omics" sciences implies that more recent learners may have less need for training in genetic concepts and newer technologies.[39] The best strategies and methodologies remain to be determined but are a critical consideration for pediatric practitioners going forward.

WHAT OF THE FUTURE FOR GENETICS IN PEDIATRIC CARE?
Genetic Testing Results Last for a Lifetime

It is likely that comprehensive genetic testing will become more common and that it will be used to assess disease risks for healthy individuals in addition to search for diagnoses in children who are symptomatic. Even if genetic testing is performed in a situation whereby it eventually turns out there is no underlying genetic diagnosis, one could argue that the genomic information generated can still provide substantial benefit in terms of screening for early cardiac and cancer morbidity and pharmacogenomic data. Genomic testing will increasingly be performed early in life so that the results are available for consultation and reinterpretation for various health-related questions and at different life stages, and pediatricians may find themselves reconsulting genetic data when new health concerns arise, or even at annual visits.

Secondary findings elucidated by ES or GS typically relate to adult-onset conditions[40] and early genetic testing can remove the autonomy of the child tested. Concerns related to the tension between parents' right to know and a child's right to an open future still exist.[41] In the future, genome-wide data may also be used to calculate polygenic risk scores (PRSs) and other statistical measures that associate the risks of individual single nucleotide polymorphisms with the likelihood of developing a disease.[42] PRSs can identify 10 to 20 times as many individuals at high risk for a condition compared with single pathogenic variants and can also modulate the effect of high-risk, monogenic alleles.[43] A multiancestral PRS for asthma could identify individuals with increased odds of developing pediatric asthma,[44] and PRSs may soon be used to identify at-risk individuals for early behavior modification strategies. A recent systematic review for evidence of clinical utility for PRSs in improving patient health did find one study that demonstrated successful use of a PRS in a risk prediction model to stratify the risk of contralateral breast cancer in women with breast cancer.[45] However, the review did not identify evidence of clinical utility, implying that further research is still needed.[10]

BRIEF SUMMARY OF IMPORTANT POINTS: OBJECTIVE POINTS TO REMEMBER

- There is a trend toward earlier implementation of more comprehensive genetic testing that covers both copy number variants and single nucleotide variants; an example of this includes the rapid ES and GS testing that are now frequently ordered in the neonatal period. This trend implies that more genetic data are likely to be available earlier in life for later use.
- Pediatricians are likely to be increasingly consulted for initiation of genetic testing and for management of genetic conditions, both rare and common.
- Shared visits between pediatricians and genetics professionals may prove to be a helpful strategy to obtain access to genomic investigations and early insurance authorization.
- The best educational strategies for genetics and genomics concepts for pediatricians are not yet well defined. Options include incorporation of teaching into daily work activities, continuing education, courses and interactive workshops, telemedicine, and participation in patient medical homes.

CLINICS CARE POINTS

- Many genetic conditions present at an early age in the pediatric patient population.
- The diagnostic yield from genetic testing is improving because of increasing use of broad testing strategies, such as microarray, ES, and GS.

- Rapid genetic testing is increasingly appropriate for critically ill patients.
- The practical benefits arising from obtaining genetic diagnosis can be substantial, including targeted treatments, disease-specific surveillance, support services, improved information for family planning, and access to clinical trials, natural history studies, and research.
- Specialized genetic tests are still warranted for some disorders despite the diagnostic strengths of broad genetic testing with ES and GS.

ACKNOWLEDGMENTS

The author is grateful to Dr Leslie Biesecker for his helpful and insightful comments.

DISCLOSURE

Dr Slavotinek is a Co-Director of the National Organization of Rare Disorders (NORD) Center of Excellence at Cincinnati Children's Hospital Medical Center.

REFERENCES

1. Lander ES, Linton LM, Birren B, et al. Initial sequencing and analysis of the human genome. Nature 2001;409:860–921, published correction appears in Nature 2001;412:565] [published correction appears in Nature 2001;411:720. Szustakowki, J [corrected to Szustakowski, J].
2. Venter JC, Adams MD, Myers EW, et al. The sequence of the human genome. Science 2001;291:1304–51, published correction appears in Science 2001;292: 1838.
3. Collins FS, Guttmacher AE. Genetics moves into the medical mainstream. JAMA 2001;286:2322–4.
4. Nurk S, Koren S, Rhie A, et al. The complete sequence of a human genome. Science 2022;376(6588):44–53.
5. Kaiser J. DNA sequencing. A plan to capture human diversity in 1000 genomes. Science 2008;319:395, published correction appears in Science 2008;319:1336.
6. Vissers LE, Veltman JA, van Kessel AG, et al. Identification of disease genes by whole genome CGH arrays. Hum Mol Genet 2005;14(Spec No. 2):R215–23.
7. Bamshad MJ, Ng SB, Bigham AW, et al. Exome sequencing as a tool for Mendelian disease gene discovery. Nat Rev Genet 2011;12. 745-5.
8. Gilissen C, Hehir-Kwa JY, Thung DT, et al. Genome sequencing identifies major causes of severe intellectual disability. Nature 2014;511:344–7.
9. Vissers LE, Gilissen C, Veltman JA. Genetic studies in intellectual disability and related disorders. Nat Rev Genet 2016;17:9–18.
10. Kumuthini J, Zick B, Balasopoulou A, et al. The clinical utility of polygenic risk scores in genomic medicine practices: a systematic review. Hum Genet 2022; 141(11):1697–704.
11. Pelter MN, Druz RS. Precision medicine: hype or hope? Trends Cardiovasc Med 2022. https://doi.org/10.1016/j.tcm.2022.11.001. S1050-1738(22)00139-6.
12. Harding B, Webber C, Ruhland L, et al. Primary care providers' lived experiences of genetics in practice. J Community Genet 2019;10:85–93.
13. Trosman JR, Weldon CB, Slavotinek A, et al. Perspectives of US private payers on insurance coverage for pediatric and prenatal exome sequencing: Results of a study from the Program in Prenatal and Pediatric Genomic Sequencing (P3EGS). Genet Med 2020;22:283–91.

14. Shah M, Selvanathan A, Baynam G, et al. Paediatric genomic testing: navigating genomic reports for the general paediatrician. J Paediatr Child Health 2022; 58:8–15.

15. French CE, Delon I, Dolling H, et al. Whole genome sequencing reveals that genetic conditions are frequent in intensively ill children. Intensive Care Med 2019; 45:627–36.

16. Kingsmore SF, Cole FS. The role of genome sequencing in neonatal intensive care units. Annu Rev Genomics Hum Genet 2022;23:427–48.

17. Smith LD, Willig LK, Kingsmore SF. Whole-exome sequencing and whole-genome sequencing in critically ill neonates suspected to have single-gene disorders. Cold Spring Harb Perspect Med 2015;6:a023168.

18. Meng L, Pammi M, Saronwala A, et al. Use of exome sequencing for infants in intensive care units: ascertainment of severe single-gene disorders and effect on medical management. JAMA Pediatr 2017;171:e173438.

19. Elliott AM, du Souich C, Lehman A, et al. RAPIDOMICS: rapid genome-wide sequencing in a neonatal intensive care unit-successes and challenges. Eur J Pediatr 2019;178:1207–18.

20. Dimmock D, Caylor S, Waldman B, et al. Project Baby Bear: Rapid precision care incorporating rWGS in 5 California children's hospitals demonstrates improved clinical outcomes and reduced costs of care. Am J Hum Genet 2021;108:1231–8.

21. Hill M, Hammond J, Lewis C, et al. Delivering genome sequencing for rapid genetic diagnosis in critically ill children: parent and professional views, experiences and challenges. Eur J Hum Genet 2020;28:1529–40.

22. Freedman AN, Wideroff L, Olson L, et al. US physicians' attitudes toward genetic testing for cancer susceptibility. Am J Med Genet 2003;120A:63–71.

23. Baynam G, Walters M, Claes P, et al. Phenotyping: targeting genotype's rich cousin for diagnosis. J Paediatr Child Health 2015;51(4):381–6. J Paediatr Child Health 2015;51:381-386.

24. Occupational outlook handbook. Washington, DC, USA: U.S. Bureau of Labor Statistics; 2017 [(accessed on 16 November 2017)].

25. Jenkins BD, Fischer CG, Polito CA, et al. The 2019 US medical genetics workforce: a focus on clinical genetics. Genet Med 2021;23:1458–64.

26. Dragojlovic N, Borle K, Kopac N, et al. The composition and capacity of the clinical genetics workforce in high-income countries: a scoping review. Genet Med 2020;22:1437–49.

27. van der Sluijs PJ, Aten E, Barge-Schaapveld DQCM, et al. Putting genome-wide sequencing in neonates into perspective. Genet Med 2019;21(5):1074–82 [Erratum in: Genet Med. 2018 Nov 21;: PMID: 30287924. Bottom of Form].

28. Muriello M. Exome and whole genome sequencing in the neonatal intensive care unit. Clin Perinatol 2022;49(1):167–79.

29. Mikat-Stevens NA, Larson IA, Tarini BA. Primary-care providers' perceived barriers to integration of genetics services: a systematic review of the literature. Genet Med 2015;17:169–76.

30. Owusu Obeng A, Fei K, Levy KD, et al. Physician-reported benefits and barriers to clinical implementation of genomic medicine: a multi-site IGNITE-network survey. J Personalized Med 2018;8:24.

31. Nisselle A, King EA, McClaren B, et al. Measuring physician practice, preparedness and preferences for genomic medicine: a national survey. BMJ Open 2021; 11:e044408. Top of Form Bottom of Form.

32. Bennett RL, French KS, Resta RG, et al. Standardized human pedigree nomenclature: update and assessment of the recommendations of the National Society of Genetic Counselors. J Genet Counsel 2008;17:424–33.
33. Hale K, Kellar-Guenther Y, McKasson S, et al. Expanding newborn screening for pompe disease in the United States: the NewSTEPs new disorders implementation project, a resource for new disorder implementation. Int J Neonatal Screen 2020;6:48.
34. Calabrò GE, Tognetto A, Mazzaccara A, et al. Capacity building of health professionals on genetics and genomics practice: evaluation of the effectiveness of a distance learning training course for Italian physicians. Front Genet 2021;12: 626685.
35. Carroll JC, Rideout AL, Wilson BJ, et al. Genetic education for primary care providers: improving attitudes, knowledge, and confidence. Can Fam Physician 2009;55:e92–9.
36. Wilkes MS, Day FC, Fancher TL, et al. Increasing confidence and changing behaviors in primary care providers engaged in genetic counselling. BMC Med Educ 2017;17:163.
37. Grol R, Grimshaw J. From best evidence to best practice: effective implementation of change in patients' care. Lancet 2003;362:1225–30.
38. Chou AF, Duncan AR, Hallford G, et al. Barriers and strategies to integrate medical genetics and primary care in underserved populations: a scoping review. J Community Genet 2021;12:291–309.
39. Hofman KJ, Tambor ES, Chase GA, et al. Physicians' knowledge of genetics and genetic tests. Acad Med 1993;68:625–32.
40. Clowes Candadai SV, Sikes MC, Thies JM, et al. Rapid clinical exome sequencing in a pediatric ICU: genetic counselor impacts and challenges. J Genet Counsel 2019;28:283–91.
41. Pereira S, Robinson JO, Gutierrez AM, et al. BabySeq Project Group. Perceived benefits, risks, and utility of newborn genomic sequencing in the BabySeq Project. Pediatrics 2019;143(Suppl 1):S6–13.
42. Khera AV, Chaffin M, Aragam KG, et al. Genome-wide polygenic scores for common diseases identify individuals with risk equivalent to monogenic mutations. Nat Genet 2018;50:1219–24.
43. Christoffersen M, Tybjærg-Hansen A. Polygenic risk scores: how much do they add? Curr Opin Lipidol 2021;32(3):157–62.
44. Namjou B, Lape M, Malolepsza E, et al. Multiancestral polygenic risk score for pediatric asthma. J Allergy Clin Immunol 2022. S0091-6749(22)00660-00661.
45. Kramer I, Hooning MJ, Mavaddat N, et al. Breast cancer polygenic risk score and contralateral breast cancer risk. Am J Hum Genet 2020;107:837–48.
46. Richards S, Aziz N, Bale S, et al. Standards and guidelines for the interpretation of sequence variants: a joint consensus recommendation of the American College of Medical Genetics and Genomics and the Association for Molecular Pathology. Genet Med 2015;17:405–24.

Genetics 101: When to Refer

Alyce Belonis, MD[a,b,]*, Sofia Saenz Ayala, MD[c]

KEYWORDS

- Genetic testing • Family history • Medical history • Inborn errors of metabolism
- Growth and developmental differences • Pediatrics

KEY POINTS

The points discussed in this manuscript serve as a resource for pediatricians to recognize the basic concepts and applications of genetics and genomics, including

- Impacts of a genetic diagnosis on patients.
- Implications of a genetic diagnosis for family members.
- Indications for referral.

INTRODUCTION

A medical genetics evaluation for a patient has the potential to be relevant to management of current signs and symptoms, provide information salient to future medical decision-making, and influence recommendations for future medical surveillance and/or genetic counseling for both the proband (patient) and biological relatives. Clinical practice in medical genetics spans a broad range of medical, developmental, and predisposition-related topics.

Each evaluation is customized to the chief complaint and, when applicable, the clinical question(s) posed by the referring medical provider. In general, evaluation includes history, with careful attention (often) paid to family history, examination, results of diagnostic studies, and consideration of further testing, both screening and diagnostic. Testing methodologies are explored in greater detail in the next article in this issue, "Clinical genetic testing options and beyond: navigating the diagnostic odyssey."

The approach to clinical management centers around careful consideration of subjective and objective information to generate a detailed phenotype, or observable trait, which drives the assessment and recommendations. This article provides contextual

[a] Division of Human Genetics, Cincinnati Children's Hospital Medical Center, 3333 Burnet Avenue, MLC 4006, Cincinnati, OH 45229, USA; [b] Department of Pediatrics, University of Cincinnati School of Medicine, Cincinnati, OH, USA; [c] Division of Human Genetics, University of Maryland Medical Center, 737 West Lombard Street, Room 199, Baltimore, MD 21201, USA
* Corresponding author. Department of Pediatrics, University of Cincinnati School of Medicine, 3333 Burnet Avenue MLC 4006, Cincinnati, OH 45229.
E-mail address: alyce.belonis@cchmc.org

Pediatr Clin N Am 70 (2023) 895–904
https://doi.org/10.1016/j.pcl.2023.05.004
0031-3955/23/© 2023 Elsevier Inc. All rights reserved.

background for, and discusses medical and developmental considerations of, common reasons for referral for the general pediatrician.

INDICATIONS FOR REFERRAL

The following sections cover different topic areas for the general pediatrician considering referral for medical genetics evaluation.

Physical Examination Findings

The physical examination serves a central role in the assessment and diagnosis of many genetic conditions. Referral for special consultation in medical genetics may center around morphology and whether findings evident on examination may indicate an underlying genetic diagnosis.

Morphology, or the development of tissue, has the capacity to inform clinical assessment, workup, diagnosis, and management recommendations (Refer to **Box 1** for a list of definitions). Although not all genetic conditions are associated with physical features that may be evident during the examination, a subset of genetic syndromes are characterized by combinations, or patterns, of physical features.

A common reason for referral for genetic evaluation is related to dysmorphology, which is a field of study, or the general subject of abnormal tissue formation. The mechanisms by which tissue does not form as expected include malformations, deformations, and disruptions.

Dysmorphology is a general descriptor about tissue formation that does not ascribe a severity, a timing, or an etiology to a malformation.[1] The study of dysmorphology has its origins in the 1950s. It has been recognized that morphological findings can be observed as isolated features in the general population and, individually, may not inform genetic assessment and diagnosis. Efforts have been made to standardize terminology to describe morphology on physical examination.[2]

A known limitation in the field of study of dysmorphology lies in the historical volume of medical literature and classic textbooks favoring clinical morphological information on individuals of Northern European descent.[2,3] More recently, publications have made an effort to include diverse populations.[4]

A morphologic evaluation by a medical geneticist can be essential to getting to, or understanding, a diagnosis for some patients who have previously received inconclusive genetic test results. In situations when a patient presents with an existing genetic

---

Box 1
Definitions

- Morphology—the development of tissue
- Dysmorphology—a field of study on, or the general subject of, abnormal tissue formation
- Phenotype—an observable trait
- Congenital anomalies—structural or functional abnormalities that are present at birth and are of prenatal origin
- Malformation—abnormal formation of tissue
- Deformation—altered morphogenesis resulting from mechanical forces
- Disruption—a destructive problem that results in breakdown of normal tissue
- Teratogen—an environmental factor that interrupts the normal development of an embryo or fetus and may result in congenital anomalies or fetal death

test report that identifies a genetic *variant of uncertain significance* (a genetic test report's classification of a finding for which the clinical significance has not yet been determined) in a gene associated with one or more phenotypes that may have a recognizable pattern of malformations, referral to medical genetics may help to elucidate whether the test result is clinically relevant to the patient.[5]

Congenital Anomalies

The presence of a severe congenital anomaly, or multiple congenital anomalies, is a common reason for referral to a medical geneticist. Congenital anomalies are structural or functional abnormalities that are present at birth and are of prenatal origin.[6]

Malformations can be intrinsic when related to an underlying genetic defect, or malformations can be extrinsic when caused by external factors. Examples of extrinsic etiologies include prenatal exposures, such as intrauterine infection, exposure to high levels of glucose (occurring in infants of diabetic mothers), and exposure to exogenous substances (teratogens). A teratogen is any agent that causes an abnormality to the fetus, following an exposure during pregnancy.[7] Teratogens can interrupt the normal development of an embryo or fetus and may result in congenital anomalies or fetal death.[6] Examples of teratogens include alcohol and medications (eg, warfarin).

Amniotic band sequence, sometimes referred to as amniotic band syndrome, is a term that describes the occurrence of a constellation of deformities and malformations that occur in a single individual, secondary to amniotic bands disrupting the physical development of a fetus, in the absence of a genetic or chromosomal etiology. The constellation of findings is unique to each individual.[8,9]

Reproductive History

The prenatal history is important to the assessment when we are concerned whether a teratogenic agent (or more than one agent) is responsible, or partially responsible, for a constellation of malformations and/or anomalies in a patient. A detailed reproductive history might reveal information that increases a suspicion for an underlying genetic disorder. These include a history of multiple miscarriages or fetal loss, which may have occurred secondary to chromosomal abnormalities or single-gene conditions (eg, incontinentia pigmenti in a male fetus); consanguinity, which may increase risk of autosomal recessive conditions; fetal birth defects; infertility, such as premature ovarian failure (eg, in fragile X-associated primary ovarian insufficiency); and carrier screening, which may reveal the risk of a specific genetic disorder in the fetus.

The effects of teratogens on the fetus are variable and depend on the teratogenic agent. For example, maternal alcohol exposure can lead to the development of fetal alcohol spectrum disorder, which is characterized by low birth weight, dysmorphic facial features, microcephaly, growth failure, and central nervous system (CNS) abnormalities. Another example of a teratogen would be an agent from the opioid class of substances, which can cause maternal complications such as preeclampsia, placental insufficiency, premature labor, and an increased risk of fetal birth defects.[10]

Growth Abnormalities

In clinic, anthropometric measurements are part of the routine physical examination and represent important indicators of the individual's growth status. Serial measurements allow for monitoring of growth parameters over time. These measurements should routinely include weight, height, and head circumference, plotted on the appropriate growth chart, recognizing that there are specific growth charts for certain conditions (eg, trisomy 21, Noonan syndrome, and others). In addition, measurements of the upper segment, lower segment, and arm span should be considered if there is a suspicion for a connective tissue disorder (eg, Marfan syndrome). Abnormalities of any of the anthropometric measurements can be an important clue to the diagnosis of growth abnormalities.

Failure to thrive (FTT) is a common sign of a wide variety of conditions, accounting for 5% to 10% of patients seen in primary care clinics and 3% to 5% of hospitalizations during infancy and early childhood.[11,12] In practical terms, FTT applies to those with weight-for-age or weight-for-length measurements that fall across (over time) two major percentiles or weight below the third percentile for sex and corrected age.[11] In evaluating FTT, screening for common etiologies that affect adequate growth and nutrition should be considered first, including an assessment of thyroid dysfunction, cystic fibrosis, anemia, and other commonly recognized pediatric chronic illnesses. If the initial workup does not yield a diagnosis, consideration for a genetic etiology is crucial as this can help predict the response to treatment and guide the evaluation for other health-related problems. The genetic differential diagnosis for FTT includes structural and numerical chromosomal abnormalities, methylation disorders, disorders of DNA repair, teratogens, inborn errors of metabolism, skeletal dysplasias, and other single-gene disorders.

Short stature is another common reason for referral. When evaluating an individual with short stature, it is important to assess whether growth failure was of prenatal or postnatal onset. Fetal growth is predominately controlled by insulin and growth factors and is affected by maternal health, nutrition, and placental function. Approximately 85% of children born small for gestational age (SGA) experience catch-up growth by 2 years of age, but the 15% remaining will have postnatal growth failure and will warrant further evaluation for a genetic etiology, including Russell-Silver syndrome, 3M syndrome, and skeletal dysplasias.[13]

During childhood, linear growth is determined by a coordinated interplay of signals that involve the hypothalamus, the anterior pituitary gland, and the growth hormone (GH) synthesis and effect via stimulation and release of the insulin-like growth factor-1 (IGF-1). Monogenic disorders affecting the GH–IGF-1 axis result in GH deficiency, either in isolation or as part of combined pituitary hormone deficiency.[14] Genetic testing in these individuals has the advantage to understand the genetic background of the condition and, in certain cases, help predict the response to treatments, including GH. In the absence of features suggestive of a specific genetic diagnosis, genetic testing should be considered in the following scenarios:

- Individuals with length/height $\leq$3 standard deviations (SD) below the mean for age
- Individuals whose length/height is $\leq$2.5 SD below the mean for age, with one or more of the additional factors:
  o Severe GH deficiency
  o Combined pituitary hormone deficiency
  o SGA without catch up growth by 2 years of age
  o Congenital anomalies or dysmorphic features
  o Intellectual disability
  o Microcephaly
- Individuals whose predicted height is $\leq$2 SD below their midparental target height.[13]

Excessive growth is the main feature of overgrowth syndromes, which are a group of disorders characterized by generalized or segmental excessive growth. Overgrowth syndromes are commonly associated with additional features, including visceromegaly and macrocephaly. Timing of presentation ranges from prenatal, with newborns who are referred for a history of being large for gestational age or macrosomic (eg, secondary to maternal diabetes or Beckwith-Wiedemann syndrome), with or without postnatal overgrowth. Accelerated growth postnatally can affect the entire body (eg, Sotos syndrome and Marfan syndrome) or can be segmental in which the excessive growth is confined to one of a few regions of the body (eg, *PIK3CA*, *PTEN* hamartoma tumor syndrome associated with macrocephaly).[15] Some of these conditions are associated with neurological dysfunction, such as cognitive impairment or autism spectrum disorder, and some may have an increased risk of cancer (embryonic tumors during infancy or carcinomas during adulthood).[16]

As mentioned above, measurement of head circumference is a critical part of a routine physical examination in every patient, particularly those who present with neurodevelopmental symptoms (eg, developmental delay, intellectual disability, autism spectrum disorder, and behavioral problems). The head circumference should be plotted in a relevant growth chart. Options for currently available growth charts for head circumference include

- CDC, for ages birth to 36 months[17]
- WHO, for ages birth to 60 months[17]
- Rollins, for ages birth to 21 years[18]

Although head circumference is a complex trait, deviations from normal head growth may be the first indication of an underlying genetic condition, warranting further evaluation with diagnostic testing, ranging from metabolic screening to neuroimaging. Microcephaly is defined as an occipitofrontal circumference (OFC) below the 3% percentile or more than 2 SD below the mean for sex, age, and ethnicity,[19,20] and it can be present at birth or develop postnatally (eg, Angelman syndrome, Rett syndrome). Macrocephaly is defined as an OFC greater than the 98th percentile and can occur as an isolated finding in familial macrocephaly or as part of a genetic syndrome without somatic overgrowth (eg, glutaric acidemia type 1, *PTEN* hamartoma tumor syndrome, neurofibromatosis type 1).[21]

Developmental Delay, Autism Spectrum Disorder, and Intellectual Disability

Some children present to clinic with a predominantly neurodevelopmental phenotype. Developmental assessment is part of the routine pediatric evaluation where a child's performance is assessed across different areas, including gross and fine motor skills, speech and language skills, cognition, and social development. Developmental delay typically refers to a child under the age of 5 years who does not meet the expected developmental milestones or learning skills for their chronological age. This can present as an isolated concern or be considered syndromic when it is identified in association with dysmorphic features, congenital anomalies, autism spectrum disorder, or epilepsy. Intellectual disability is characterized by an impairment in cognitive ability and adaptive functioning and is assessed in school-age, and older, children.[22]

Genetic testing is an important diagnostic tool for the evaluation of neurodevelopmental disorders. Identifying the genetic basis of an individual's developmental delay, autism spectrum disorder, or intellectual disability provides essential information about prognosis, individualized needs, and reproductive risk. There is a body of evidence that supports consideration of the following methodologies: chromosomal microarray analysis, exome and genome sequencing, and *FMR1* CGG repeat analysis.[23,24] A recent study demonstrated that the cumulative diagnostic yield is greater than 50% for individuals with global developmental delay and intellectual disability and greater than 25% for individuals whose primary neurodevelopmental diagnosis is autism spectrum disorder.[23]

Inborn Errors of Metabolism

Another common reason for a genetics referral is a suspected inborn error of metabolism (IEM). These group of disorders are heterogenous and involve failure of the metabolic pathways involved in either the breakdown or storage of carbohydrates, fatty acids, and proteins. IEMs are individually rare, but as a group, they are relatively common and can present at any age. Although newborn screening has now become widely available and many individuals are being identified with an IEM before the onset of symptoms, there are some disorders that are not included on the newborn screen. The conditions screened for vary from state to state (see Chapter 11).

Having a high index of suspicion for the possibility of an IEM is critical for early detection and rapid intervention to minimize neurological sequalae and prevent death. Several groups of inherited metabolic disorders, most notably the organic acidemias, urea cycle defects, and certain disorders of amino acid metabolism, classically present shortly after birth with metabolic decompensation that leads to life-threatening encephalopathy, due to accumulation of metabolites that have CNS toxicity.[25] In these individuals, initial symptoms of lethargy and poor feeding overlap with the presenting symptoms of sepsis. The high acuity and overlap with sepsis pose a challenge for pediatricians. However, not all IEMs present acutely in the first days of life; subtle symptoms of IEMs can become evident in later childhood, adolescence, or adulthood.

A detailed history is important in the evaluation of a child with a suspected IEM. This includes dietary history, with emphasis on any dietary restrictions (eg, restricted protein or carbohydrate intake), special diet (eg, high-protein diet, any dietary supplements), and feeding pattern including fasting periods. Other aspects of the medical history that might be relevant include FTT, history of frequent hospital admissions, persistent vomiting, seizures, developmental delay, and hypotonia. It is important to get a thorough family history although a negative family history does not exclude the possibility of an IEM. A history of a full sibling who had sudden infant death should raise the clinical suspicion for an undiagnosed fatty acid oxidation disorder.

Elements of the physical examination that may be relevant in determining whether to refer a patient for medical genetics evaluation include, but are not limited to,

- Dysmorphic features (eg, coarse facies in mucopolysaccharidosis, peroxisomal disorders)
- Specific odors (eg, sweaty feet in isovaleric acidemia, maple syrup in maple syrup urine disease, musty odor in phenylketonuria)
- Level of alertness, neurological signs (eg, abnormal movement, abnormal tone, and reflexes)
- Organomegaly (eg, splenomegaly in Gaucher disease and Niemann-Pick disease)
- Differences in skin pigmentation (eg, generalized hyperpigmentation in Wilson disease)
- Cardiac dysfunction (eg, cardiomyopathy in several long-chain fatty acid oxidation disorders and Fabry disease).

It is important to note that unexpected odors should be considered within an overall clinical context when considering referral for medical genetics evaluation.

Medical History

Beyond malformations and deformations, an individual's personal medical history may be the central reason for referral to medical genetics. Medical history can be either straightforward and encompass a single organ system, such as a past medical history of sensorineural hearing loss (SNHL), or it may be more complex and involve multiple organ systems. Complicating these considerations is the knowledge that history of a single medical condition could either end up being truly self-contained, with respect to the organ system, or it could be the earliest manifestation of a genetic condition characterized by the involvement of multiple organ systems. SNHL, for example, may occur in isolation and therefore be characterized as "nonsyndromic," or it could be the first clinically apparent finding for a patient with a diagnosis of Usher syndrome, which also involves retinal dystrophy that develops at an age beyond the patient's age at the time of initial evaluation for hearing loss. A failed hearing screen, which raises clinical suspicion for a diagnosis of SNHL, might be the first clinically apparent finding in a patient who has an underlying diagnosis of a mitochondrial disorder, which can affect many organ systems and can be, for some patients, life-limiting. The aforementioned examples related to SNHL highlight the importance of identifying a genetic etiology early, as an etiology can be crucial to establishing developmental and medical expectations that would provide context for future medical decision-making.

A medical genetics evaluation and workup for an individual with either an apparently straightforward or a complex medical history can provide key information for health (physical and psychosocial) and developmental outcomes. A unifying genetic diagnosis could:

- Serve as a foundation around which a clinical framework can be designed to guide future medical management and/or surveillance. On occasion, a specific genetic test result is the determining factor that provides an opportunity to participate in a particular clinical trial or receive specific therapy for their medical condition
- Provide relevant information that could inform a change in patient/family goals of care in the acute setting
- Help caregivers develop expectations for future developmental trajectory and plan for future developmental interventions
- Result in overall cost-of-care savings in certain inpatient settings (eg, the intensive care unit)[26]
- Identify other biological relatives who may be at risk
- Inform genetic counseling for patients and family members
- Resolve the uncertainty that patients and/or families experienced before knowing the underlying reason for their medical history
- Inform recurrence risk counseling for the individual, as well as the individual's biological parents

Medical conditions may have an underlying genetic etiology. Such examples include, but are not limited to, conditions that present with the following symptoms:

- Limitations in hearing (eg, SNHL)
- Low vision (eg, retinal dystrophy)
- Impaired muscle movement, or abnormal muscle tone (eg, neuromuscular disorders)
- Impaired cardiac function (eg, cardiomyopathy)
- Frequent lung infections (eg, cystic fibrosis, primary ciliary dyskinesia, or specific immunodeficiency)
- Disorders of the skin (eg, ichthyosis).

Sometimes, medical conditions can occur in the setting of an underlying genetic diagnosis that may also be characterized by dysmorphic features, malformations, and/or developmental differences. One such example includes Williams syndrome; individuals with Williams syndrome can have developmental delay, intellectual disability, and medical problems that span multiple organ systems, such as cardiac malformations including supravalvular aortic stenosis, hypothyroidism, hypertension, and hypercalcemia/hypercalciuria.

Hereditary Cancer Predisposition

Hereditary cancer predisposition is another category of conditions for which genetics referral should be considered. Such an evaluation can help to characterize an individual's risk of developing tumors or cancer at some point during their lifetime. Rarely, infants are born with a tumor, or have a more specific cancer diagnosis at the time of birth (eg, hepatoblastoma). Most commonly, they are referred because their individual medical history, and/or their family history, suggests that there may be a higher risk of developing tumors or cancer than the risk for the general population.

A prominent reason for wanting to determine whether an individual has an underlying tumor predisposition syndrome is to identify salient recommendations for present-day and future medical surveillance. The purpose of surveillance is to be able to identify early signs of cancer, so that the condition can be treated early on in the disease course.

The other potential benefits of referral for hereditary cancer predisposition evaluation overlap with many of those listed in the previous section on referrals due to straightforward or complex medical history. In addition, there can be clinical situations for which knowing the underlying genetic mechanism will inform management. For example, a known genetic mechanism could be a determining factor in a decision to avoid radiation therapy for a particular tumor type.

The age of the patient is relevant in medical genetics evaluation for hereditary cancer predisposition. If a pediatric patient, who has not yet reached the age of majority, is being referred on the basis of family history only, without any personal past medical history of signs or symptoms of a tumor predisposition syndrome, one important consideration is to take into account the youngest recommended age at which specific screening protocols are recommended. In general, for patients who may not have yet attained the age of majority but are expected to have the capacity to consent to genetics evaluation after they reach the age of majority, and where family history does not suggest that the individual needs to receive specific surveillance prior to the age of majority, it is not recommended to override the individual's future potential autonomy by sending genetic testing before the age of majority. This situation is ideally addressed through genetic counseling. There may be limited, individualized situations for which predictive genetic testing should be considered prior to the age of majority.[27–29] It is still worthwhile to consider referral for pediatric patient who has only a specific family history, regardless of the expected age when surveillance would need to start, because sometimes, patients and families may find it helpful to have an informed conversation about what to expect. An office visit can provide the needed space for patients and caregivers to discuss the complexity of the different considerations around whether the interests of the patient regarding genetic testing for adult-onset conditions, even when a pediatric patient has not yet reached the age of majority, outweigh the potential harms.

Family History of Confirmed Genetic Diagnosis

These include one or more family members with a known history of intellectual disability, developmental delay, a specific genetic diagnosis, or a birth defect, which might increase the recurrence risk within a family. It is also important to document if one or more family members had an early death, or adult-onset health condition like cardiovascular disease, dementia, or cancer, particularly if onset is early in adulthood.

SUMMARY

The aforementioned topics discussed in this article, encompassing themes related to developmental history, medical history, and family history, provide a broad range of examples of common reasons for referral for pediatric patients. All patients have unique aspects of their histories, any of which might serve as the key to understanding the core issue(s) at hand, and that possibility makes it challenging to create a precise roadmap or algorithm for referral that could be generalized to any specific patient. For cases for which a question remains about whether medical genetics referral is appropriate, it may be worthwhile to consider discussing the case of your patient with your local (or regional) medical genetics consultant prior to deciding on whether to initiate a referral.

CLINICS CARE POINTS

- Medical genetics evaluations can provide valuable clinical information that can inform present and future management, surveillance, and/or prognosis for patients of all ages who have medical and/or developmental histories consistent with a genetic etiology

- Family history can provide crucial information that may impact genetic counseling

- Anthropomorphic measurements and dysmorphology examinations play a central role in guiding genetics workup and management recommendations

- A genetic or teratogenic etiology should be considered in the evaluation of a patient with dysmorphic features, other concerning examination findings, abnormal growth, abnormal development, and/or complex medical history

DISCLOSURE

There are no relevant conflicts of interest to disclose.

REFERENCES

1. Smith DW. Dysmorphology (teratology). J Pediatr 1966;69(6):1150–69.
2. Allanson JE, Biesecker LG, Carey JC, et al. Elements of morphology: Introduction. Am J Med Genet 2009;149A(1):2–5.
3. Muenke M, Adeyemo A, Kruszka P. An electronic atlas of human malformation syndromes in diverse populations. Genet Med 2016;18(11):1085–7.
4. Kruszka P, Tekendo-Ngongang C, Muenke M. Diversity and dysmorphology. Curr Opin Pediatr 2019;31(6):702–7.
5. Hurst ACE, Robin NH. Dysmorphology in the Era of Genomic Diagnosis. J Personalized Med 2020;10(1):18.
6. Organization WH, Control CfD, Prevention. Birth defects surveillance: a manual for programme managers. In:2020.
7. Genetic A. The New York-Mid-Atlantic Consortium for G, Newborn Screening S. Genetic Alliance Monographs and Guides (series): Understanding Genetics: A New York, Mid-Atlantic Guide for Patients and Health Professionals (book). In: Understanding genetics: a New York, mid-atlantic guide for patients and health

professionals. Washington (DC): Genetic Alliance Copyright © 2008, Genetic Alliance; 2009.

8. Seeds JW, Cefalo RC, Herbert WN. Amniotic band syndrome. Am J Obstet Gynecol 1982;144(3):243–8.

9. Gandhi M, Rac MWF, McKinney J. Amniotic Band Sequence. Am J Obstet Gynecol 2019;221(6):B5–6.

10. Cleary B, Loane M, Addor MC, et al. Methadone, Pierre Robin sequence and other congenital anomalies: case-control study. Arch Dis Child Fetal Neonatal Ed 2020;105(2):151–7.

11. Schwartz ID. Failure to thrive: an old nemesis in the new millennium. Pediatr Rev 2000;21(8):257–64, quiz 264.

12. Daniel M, Kleis L, Cemeroglu AP. Etiology of failure to thrive in infants and toddlers referred to a pediatric endocrinology outpatient clinic. Clin Pediatr (Phila) 2008;47(8):762–5.

13. Dauber A, Rosenfeld RG, Hirschhorn JN. Genetic evaluation of short stature. J Clin Endocrinol Metab 2014;99(9):3080–92.

14. David A, Hwa V, Metherell LA, et al. Evidence for a continuum of genetic, phenotypic, and biochemical abnormalities in children with growth hormone insensitivity. Endocr Rev 2011;32(4):472–97.

15. Manor J, Lalani SR. Overgrowth Syndromes-Evaluation, Diagnosis, and Management. Front Pediatr 2020;8:574857.

16. Brioude F, Toutain A, Giabicani E, et al. Overgrowth syndromes - clinical and molecular aspects and tumour risk. Nat Rev Endocrinol 2019;15(5):299–311.

17. Grummer-Strawn LM, Reinold C, Krebs NF. Use of World Health Organization and CDC growth charts for children aged 0-59 months in the United States. MMWR Recomm Rep (Morb Mortal Wkly Rep) 2010;59(Rr-9):1–15.

18. Rollins JD, Collins JS, Holden KR. United States head circumference growth reference charts: birth to 21 years. J Pediatr 2010;156(6):907–13.e902.

19. Opitz JM, Holt MC. Microcephaly: general considerations and aids to nosology. J Craniofac Genet Dev Biol 1990;10(2):175–204.

20. Hanzlik E, Gigante J. Microcephaly. Children 2017;4(6).

21. Sniderman A. Abnormal head growth. Pediatr Rev 2010;31(9):382–4.

22. Bellman M, Byrne O, Sege R. Developmental assessment of children. BMJ 2013; 346:e8687.

23. Savatt JM, Myers SM. Genetic Testing in Neurodevelopmental Disorders. Front Pediatr 2021;9:526779.

24. Manickam K, McClain MR, Demmer LA, et al. Exome and genome sequencing for pediatric patients with congenital anomalies or intellectual disability: an evidence-based clinical guideline of the American College of Medical Genetics and Genomics (ACMG). Genet Med 2021;23(11):2029–37.

25. Burton BK. Inborn errors of metabolism in infancy: a guide to diagnosis. Pediatrics 1998;102(6):E69.

26. Dimmock D, Caylor S, Waldman B, et al. Project Baby Bear: Rapid precision care incorporating rWGS in 5 California children's hospitals demonstrates improved clinical outcomes and reduced costs of care. Am J Hum Genet 2021;108(7):1231–8.

27. Ross LF, Saal HM, David KL, et al. Technical report: Ethical and policy issues in genetic testing and screening of children. Genet Med 2013;15(3):234–45.

28. Ethical and policy issues in genetic testing and screening of children. Pediatrics 2013;131(3):620–2.

29. Garrett JR, Lantos JD, Biesecker LG, et al. Rethinking the "open future" argument against predictive genetic testing of children. Genet Med 2019;21(10):2190–8.

Panels, Exomes, Genomes, and More—Finding the Best Path Through the Diagnostic Odyssey

Arthur L. Lenahan, MD, MPH[a], Audrey E. Squire, MS, CGC[a],
Danny E. Miller, MD, PhD[a,b,*]

KEYWORDS

• Genetic testing • Short read sequencing • Long read sequencing • Rare disease

KEY POINTS

• Clinical genetics is a rapidly evolving field as new technologies are introduced, and new gene-phenotype associations are made.

• A precise genetic diagnosis allows individuals and their families to potentially receive more accurate information about the prognosis and recurrence risk of a genetic condition, as well as information regarding future screening or age-related risks.

• Negative or nondiagnostic genetic testing results do not entirely rule out an underlying genetic etiology. There may be limitations to the technology used, as even a "comprehensive" exomes and genomes do not capture all possible mechanisms. Additionally, our understanding of human genetics is incomplete, and most patients with nondiagnostic testing are reevaluated in the future.

• Emerging genetic testing approaches include but are not limited to genome-wide methylation analysis, long-read DNA sequencing, and RNA sequencing, which have the goal of increasing the rate of genetic diagnoses and ending the "diagnostic odyssey" for many individuals and their families.

The evaluation of individuals with a suspected genetic disorder has evolved rapidly over the past 10 years with the introduction of new testing modalities, such as exome sequencing (ES). These new technologies are beneficial as they offer the possibility of precise genetic diagnoses, which can inform screening guidelines, provide critical prognostic information, and permit informed discussions about recurrence risks.[1] Because of the rapid pace of change in terms of both diagnostic options and our

[a] Division of Genetic Medicine, Department of Pediatrics, University of Washington and Seattle Children's Hospital, 4800 Sand Point Way, Seattle, WA 98105, USA; [b] Department of Laboratory Medicine and Pathology, University of Washington, Seattle, WA, USA
* Corresponding author. 1959 Pacific Street, Seattle, WA 98195.
E-mail address: dm1@uw.edu

Pediatr Clin N Am 70 (2023) 905–916
https://doi.org/10.1016/j.pcl.2023.06.001
0031-3955/23/© 2023 Elsevier Inc. All rights reserved.

knowledge about the molecular underpinnings of most genetic disorders, it can be challenging to stay up-to-date with new testing methods and recommendations. In addition, new complex testing modalities have a higher likelihood of identifying uncertain or secondary results in situations where there is a high suspicion of a genetic disorder.

Here, we review commonly used clinical genetic tests and their limitations, including karyotype, single nucleotide polymorphism (SNP) microarrays, next-generation sequencing panels, comprehensive studies such as exome and genome sequencing, and methylation-based testing. Despite a great deal of advancement in the sensitivity and accuracy of commonly used clinical tests, difficulties remain in terms of interpreting uncertain results or how to proceed after negative testing. In addition, we will discuss new technologies that are either infrequently used on a clinical basis today or are still being evaluated in the research setting, and how these may be used for individuals with negative or uncertain results.

CURRENT TESTING MODALITIES

Precise genetic diagnoses are sought for multiple reasons. For example, a family with a critically ill neonate may seek additional information when considering goals of care, or a treatment team may use the information to recommend a specific medication. Short-term benefits to the early identification of genetic disorders include earlier intervention in disorders with progressive risk, such as cardiac and cancer predisposition syndromes, and improved ability to mitigate episodic crises, as may be seen in metabolic disorders. Long-term benefits include informed counseling regarding recurrence risk, improved preventive care with surveillance, involvement of families in support communities, and potential for involvement in research, which may lead to better understanding of the natural histories and management of rare disorders.[2,3]

Before discussing specific types of tests that can be ordered, it is important to consider possible results of genetic testing. Broadly, results are either: positive, in that the underlying etiology for the patient's features was identified; negative, in that it was not; or uncertain, meaning a change was identified, but its relationship to the phenotype is unclear. Each finding is classified along a spectrum, ranging from a "benign" or "likely benign" to a "variant of uncertain significance" (VUS) to "likely pathogenic" (LP) or "pathogenic" variant (**Table 1**). Formal classification criteria has been published by the American College of Medical Genetics.[4] Diagnostic results, often termed "positive," where an underlying causative pathogenic or likely pathogenic variant was identified, is typically the goal of genetic testing. Results must always be reviewed by the ordering clinician to ensure they indeed explain the clinical phenotype. Testing laboratories may be operating with limited information about the individual being tested, and it is possible that a positive result may not fully explain the individual's phenotype or future risk of developing features. Nondiagnostic, or negative results, are situations in which no or only benign findings were identified. VUSs can be challenging to interpret as they mean a change was detected that may be associated with the clinical presentation, but data are lacking to more definitively determine whether the change is indeed disease-causing.

Chromosomal Approaches

A common first-line genetic testing approach is chromosomal analysis, which we define to include either karyotype and/or microarray. A karyotype can be used to detect both differences in chromosome number and to identify large structural changes, such as translocations, large inversions, or large deletions or duplications.

Table 1
Variant classification

Variant Type	Definition	Supporting Evidence	Follow up Recommendations
Benign	No evidence of genetic etiology causative of symptoms.	Many individuals carry this variant in the population without increased risk of clinical features (>5% of population in exome databases). Little to no evidence of impact on protein function in vitro.	None
Likely benign VUS	Variant cannot be definitively ruled out as a genetic factor, but no or little evidence to support association. Typically represents normal genetic variation.	Family members carry the variant without evidence of disorder. Variant includes a site not adjacent to regions known to cause functional impact on protein.	None
VUS with moderate evidence of pathogenicity	Mix of evidence for and against pathogenicity. Unclear result with need for clinical correlation.	Combination of supporting features of both likely benign and likely pathogenic VUSs. Variant is located in a mutational hot spot, or a site well known to impact protein function.	Genetic counseling recommended. Consider family member testing or more comprehensive testing as discussed. Recommend follow up with genetics every 1–3 years for the reclassification of variant if clinical suspicion.
Likely pathogenic	Variant not previously described to be pathogenic but weight of evidence supports relationship to clinical features.	Few individuals in population carry variant. Variant is new (de novo) in the affected individual, or family members are affected who also carry the variant. Variant site is adjacent to or includes a region or base pair known to cause functional impact. Evidence in vitro for functional impact of variant on protein function.	Genetic counseling recommended. Manage as pathogenic if clinical reasoning supports this diagnosis.
Pathogenic	Known association between variant and clinical features ("positive" result) based on a well-defined body of evidence.	See likely pathogenic.	Genetic counseling recommended. Prevention and treatment as indicated for disorder.

Abbreviation: VUS, variant of uncertain significance.
Adapted from Richards et al.[4]

Karyotype is often used to evaluate for aneuploidy in patients with high pretest probability of a trisomy such as trisomy 13, 18, or 21, or to evaluate for sex chromosome differences such as in suspected cases of Turner syndrome or in the setting of ambiguous genitalia. Overall, the use of karyotype in neonates has been declining as prenatal chromosomal screening, such as cell-free fetal DNA (cffDNA) testing, has expanded.[5] Individuals in which cffDNA identifies an aneuploidy, or some other large chromosome change. Because cffDNA is a screening test individuals need to have a karyotype to confirm the findings.[6] One disadvantage of karyotypes is the low resolution, as it is only able to detect the presence of large changes at the chromosomal level such as deletions, duplications, structural abnormalities (such as a ring chromosome), and translocations greater than 5-10 megabase (Mb) pairs.[7]

A chromosomal microarray (often called a "SNP array") provides higher resolution than a karyotype, and can identify smaller imbalances of genetic material (deletions or duplications) than a karyotype.[8] Current microarray technology uses a high volume of probes for common single nucleotide polymorphisms (SNPs) distributed along the chromosome in order to identify changes in copy number (ie, the number of copies of a given gene). Although much more sensitive for imbalances, a microarray does not "visualize" the chromosomes, and will therefore not detect gross-level abnormalities such as a ring chromosome, inversions, or a balanced translocation where there is no change in copy number.

Regions with loss of heterozygosity (LOH), or the presence of the same genetic material on both chromosomes, may also be detected with a SNP array. When LOH is observed, depending on the pattern, the clinician should suspect either shared ancestry/consanguinity between parents, or uniparental disomy (UPD). UPD occurs when both copies of that chromosome or region came from one parent (specifically, isodisomy).[9] In an individual with a compelling phenotype regions with LOH might be more closely evaluated to determine if any high-priority genes of interest that follow a recessive inheritance pattern are within the region.

As a category, chromosomal abnormalities, including microdeletion/duplication syndromes, are a frequent cause of congenital anomalies and developmental delay. It is important to remember that small deletions or duplications, such as those encompassing a single exon, may still be missed by standard microarray and warrant further testing for the detection of deletions within genes or broader testing via next-generation sequencing.[10]

Targeted Approaches and Panel Testing

Broadly, sequencing approaches include a number of different techniques that can determine the nucleotide sequence of a specific genomic region (such as an exon), an individual gene, or sets of genes known to be associated with a common set of physical features or symptoms (commonly referred to as a panel). Next-generation sequencing (NGS) or short-read sequencing, is commonly used in these situations to identify single nucleotide changes or small insertions or deletions in genes of interest.

Single-gene testing with an NGS panel may be used in cases with high pretest suspicion for a specific single-gene disorder, such as a child with a biochemical profile that suggests methylmalonic acidemia, or a family history suggestive of an adult-onset cancer predisposition syndrome. Beyond targeted examples such as these, there is wide variability in how genetic testing panels are used. Over the last decade, there has been a rapid increase in the number of available panels from private laboratories, each with an ever-expanding catalog of included genes. This clustered approach to targeted sequencing has resulted in wide variability between tests, depending on the panel or the laboratory. For example, a panel of genes associated with autism and intellectual disability might range from 50 to more than 2,500 single genes, with some labs not undertaking analysis for copy-number variation.

In practice, use rates of panels vary significantly between specialties and institutions, with mixed evidence around the cost-effectiveness of this approach. The utility of gene panels is currently decreasing as the size of gene panels increases, since their marginal utility diminishes compared to comprehensive sequencing methods. Indeed, a recent study comparing rates of inconclusive results between gene panels and comprehensive methods in a large dataset found that panels identify more VUSs than comprehensive testing (32% versus 23%, respectively), calling into question the utility of panels moving forward.[11]

Comprehensive Approaches: Exome and Genome Sequencing

Exome (ES) and genome sequencing (GS) represent the most comprehensive approaches to genetic testing available, and ideally include parents or siblings as comparators. Until recently, this technology was reserved for the most complex unsolved cases, but with increased availability and utility, ES and GS are quickly being applied to clinical settings. ES, first introduced in clinical diagnostics in 2011, sequences the 1–2% of the human genome that codes for proteins (ie, exons), and currently evaluates about 21,000 genes.[12] Because the DNA sequence of a gene is mostly non-coding sequence known as an intron it is important to keep in mind that the entire sequence of each gene is not analyzed, thus pathogenic changes in introns which may affect the function of the gene or nearby regulatory regions which may affect the expression of the gene may be missed. Copy number variation may or may not be included, and ES does not analyze other disease-causing mechanisms such as repeat expansions or methylation abnormalities. Alternatively, short-read genome sequencing (srGS), captures all regions, allowing analysis of intronic and regulatory regions.[13] Similar to ES, GS data can be re-interpreted, either clinically after a period of time or on a research basis, to identify new gene-phenotype associations or identify variants missed by previous analysis.

Exome sequencing has already had a large impact on the clinical genetics evaluation and workup, with benefits to both the provider and patient/family. As of 2021, the American College of Medical Genetics (ACMG) recommends ES as a first-line genetic test for individuals with multiple congenital anomalies and/or intellectual disability.[14] Notably, rapid ES and srGS have found utility in the critical care setting, such as the NICU and PICU.[15,16] Multiple studies have demonstrated that in this specific patient population a precise genetic diagnosis could inform both treatment choices and decisions regarding goals of care.[17] Furthermore, there is emerging evidence that GS has an overall higher diagnostic yield than ES with comparable rates of inconclusive results.[11,13]

Because ES and srGS are broad tests, it is important to consider that the data may include information in genes unrelated to the patient's phenotype or reason for testing. The ACMG has published a list of recommended genes determined to be of clear medical significance, as each has associated screening or management guidelines.[18] These are referred to as "secondary findings," and examples include genes associated with cancer predisposition syndromes, cardiac arrhythmias and inborn errors of metabolism. Families undergoing ES or GS should receive pre-test counseling to discuss possible implications of these results as well as the option to opt-out of secondary findings.

Limitations to both srGS and ES include increased cost and an increased burden of uncertain findings when compared to a karyotype or a microarray. ES specifically can only evaluate intronic variants near exons, and thus may miss deep intronic variants that alter splicing. Both srGS and ES may have difficulty detecting certain structural variants such as inversions, depending on how the data is analyzed, and not all laboratories are validated to analyze the ES data for copy number variation; thus, the ordering clinician needs to be aware of these differences and limitations during test selection. Despite these complexities, there is increasing evidence that a broad approach to clinical testing, such as with ES, is a cost-effective first-line approach and thus is becoming more widely supported by payers and institutions.[14]

In cases where ES or srGS results are negative, there are a few important points to consider. First, both may not fully cover or sequence-specific genes of interest, or the coverage may be too low to fully evaluate. Some variants are inherently difficult to detect, such as mosaic variants. Depth of sequencing coverage is important to consider as higher degrees of coverage improve the level of confidence in detected variants. Target coverage varies between laboratories, thus, if there is a question of mosaicism, or concern for coverage of a specific gene, the ordering provider should reach out to the lab for clarification. Some studies have shown a "false negative rate" for variants missed by ES of around 2-3%.[19] The question of whether srGS has a significantly higher yield than ES remains open. Existing studies have demonstrated a 5–21% increased diagnostic yield of srGS over ES, but it remains unclear as to whether this difference will be sustained in larger more carefully controlled studies.[20]

Testing for Imprinting Disorders and Repeat Expansions

Several types of genetic changes are difficult to detect with the modalities discussed above. These include imprinting disorders and repeat expansions. Imprinting disorders result from errors in the epigenetic markers on DNA termed methylation, which affect the expression of genes, but these marks do not change the underlying DNA sequence. Specialized testing is needed if there is high clinical suspicion of an imprinting disorder. Common disorders caused by imprinting errors include Beckwith-Wiedemann syndrome, Prader-Willi syndrome, Angelman syndrome, and Silver-Russel syndrome.[21] Repeat expansions are also difficult to detect due to the sequencing method, which reads DNA in 100 to 150 base pair fragments. To accomplish this, DNA is first fragmented followed by in silico regeneration and alignment, which can make it difficult to reliably characterize long lengths of repeated DNA. Common repeat expansion disorders include Huntington disease, Fragile-X syndrome, Friedreich's ataxia, and the spinocerebellar ataxias, among others.[22]

NAVIGATING THE DIAGNOSTIC ODYSSEY

The approach to clinical genetic testing has changed over the past 20 years. This is in part due to availability, and studies that have demonstrated the benefit of specific tests in specific patient populations, such as the benefit of rapid ES in the critical care setting.[16] In addition, society guidelines have changed over time, shifting the recommended first-line diagnostic tests for certain conditions, such as intellectual disability.[14] Because of these shifts it can be challenging for the non-genetics professional to select the best test for a specific phenotype. Later in discussion is a general guide for clinicians who are considering ordering genetic testing and important points to consider when ordering testing.

Congenital Anomalies, Intellectual Disability, or Developmental Delay

Genetic testing is commonly performed for patients with developmental delay, dysmorphic facial features, and poor feeding/growth. These may be nonspecific features and not generally tied to a single organ system, where targeted testing would have a poor overall yield. In such cases, either a SNP array or ES is typically the first test of choice, with ES sent to a lab that can also perform CNV analysis being the likely highest yield option. The clinician should consider whether the individual has significant malformations or striking dysmorphic features that might suggest aneuploidy, and thus a karyotype would be a reasonable place to start.

SNP array is often used as a first test for individuals with developmental delay either with or without other congenital anomalies. In 2021, the ACMG released an evidence-based clinical practice guideline on the use of ES or srGS in pediatric patients with congenital anomalies, developmental delay, or intellectual disability that found ES or srGS has a higher diagnostic yield and may be more cost-effective than other testing modalities.[14] For neonates in the NICU with congenital anomalies, multiple studies have shown the benefit of rapid ES or srGS. For example, a recent study found an overall diagnostic yield of 46% (28/61) in a cohort of NICU neonates with pathology not explained by prematurity or a clear environmental trigger.[3] The utility of srGS as a first-line strategy in this population is being explored, with an estimated 30-40% overall yield.[2] However, srGS has not been shown to be superior to ES in the NICU at this time.

The workup for individuals with nonspecific presentations that do not fit a well-described syndrome remains challenging. Often providers may start with a gene panel guided by one or more elements of the phenotype, but these may only be indicated in specific situations. A panel is likely a good choice in a situation where an inborn error of metabolism is suspected based on biochemical testing, with the yield as high as 64% in one study.[23] For some phenotypes, ES has shown superiority over panel testing. In individuals with epilepsy, for example, a recent study found the yield of ES to be 45% compared to 23% for a standard panel.[24]

Methylation Disorders and Repeat Expansions

As mentioned above, many commonly ordered genetic tests such as karyotype, SNP array, or ES are unlikely to capture changes associated with imprinting disorders or repeat expansions. Certain symptom sets should prompt the inclusion of specialized testing either in parallel or as a reflex, if prior testing is negative. For example, Prader-Willi syndrome, which is caused by the loss of paternally inherited genes on the long arm of chromosome 15, is characterized by early hypotonia and feeding difficulty, which progresses to generalized developmental delays and hyperphagia later in childhood. Evaluation is by methylation studies, which can capture both copy number variants affecting the imprinting locus and epigenetic changes.[25] Similarly, Beckwith-Wiedemann syndrome, characterized by features that include macrosomia, macro-glossia, hemi hyperplasia, omphalocele, and hyperinsulinism, is associated with an imprinting defect on the short arm of chromosome 11 in about half of the cases. Because of this specialized evaluation, including methylation studies are required for the molecular diagnosis.[26]

Fragile X syndrome (FXS) is an X-linked disorder associated with developmental delay, intellectual disability, autism, and features of connective tissue disease such as joint laxity and flat feet caused by CGG expansion in *FMR1*. Early reports overestimated the prevalence of FXS, now suspected to be around 14:100,000.[27] Previously, trinucleotide repeat analysis was sent as part of first-line workup for generalized developmental delay. Given the reduced population prevalence, this specialized testing may be sent after normal exome sequencing and SNP array, neither of which can evaluate for expansion of the repeat.

Family Members of an Affected Individual

Establishing a genetic diagnosis may have extensive implications for families of affected individuals, and genetic testing for the biological relatives is performed in multiple scenarios. Comprehensive testing with both ES or srGS routinely includes parents and/or siblings for comparison, meaning that the inheritance of each variant is determined with the proband's results, often allowing for additional interpretation. Multiple studies have shown the benefit of including comparator samples in analysis. If relatives aren't included in initial testing, targeted follow-up testing is often recommended, and some commercial laboratories offer familial testing at no-charge.

In the setting of a VUS, the inheritance of the variant can sometimes help interpret its pathogenicity. For example, if a VUS is identified in an autosomal dominant gene and neither parent is a carrier, meaning that it arose new, or *de novo*, for the patient, clinical suspicion regarding the variant's pathogenicity might increase. Conversely, if one or both parents do have the same VUS, and are otherwise healthy and unaffected, suspicion of pathogenicity may decrease. Of note, testing for a variant of uncertain significance is not typically performed in order to dictate relatives' medical management.

If a diagnostic pathogenic or likely pathogenic variant is identified, the inheritance possibilities include that it arose *de novo* in this patient, versus it was inherited from one or both parents, depending on the gene's inheritance pattern. The *de novo* rate varies widely between individual genes. If the underlying variant(s) were inherited, the patient's parent(s) may have their own healthcare management to address, and additional relatives may also be at-risk. The inheritance of a variant also guides accurate recurrent risk counseling for the patient's parents and family.

Given the implications of genetic diagnoses for families, both medically and psychosocially, focused counseling is important. Possible outcomes and secondary findings should always be discussed prior to ordering testing, and some families are additionally concerned about legal implications. The current Genetic Information Nondisclosure Act (GINA) is designed to protect families from increased insurance costs incurred by genetic testing, but there are known loopholes, including private life insurance.[28] GINA has not yet been tested in court. Of note, research suggests an overall positive psychological impact of definitive molecular diagnosis for families, with an estimated 81% of families reporting that genome sequencing was useful whether diagnostic or nondiagnostic.[29]

Next Steps After a Negative Clinical Evaluation

Cases sometimes arise with negative clinical testing where suspicion for a genetic disorder remains high. In these scenarios, the best path forward is unclear. Careful re-evaluation of the phenotype and revisiting family history may uncover additional clues that could drive variant interpretation or test selection. Follow-up visits with the individual may reveal new symptoms not previously described that may point to a specific gene or pathway. If ES had been previously performed, reanalysis after 12-18 months may allow for the assessment of new gene-phenotype associations that have been discovered since the test was performed initially. Reanalysis has been shown to be high-yield.[30] In those cases with negative testing, referral to a group working on the specific phenotype or a large consortium such as the Undiagnosed Diseases Network may be considered.[31]

THE FUTURE: NEW AND EMERGING GENETIC MODALITIES

Several new and emerging technologies have the potential to impact current practices in clinical genetic testing and offer additional options for those individuals without a precise genetic diagnosis. These include RNA sequencing, methylation profiling, optical genome mapping (OGM), and long-read sequencing (LRS). RNA-sequencing and methylation profiling can be ordered on a clinical basis at the time of this writing, while optical mapping and long-read sequencing cannot. RNA-sequencing can be used to identify differences in mRNA structure, or gene expression.[32,33] This can be done to look at a specific gene of interest or more broadly a profile of all genes expressed in the tissue evaluated. As an example, RNA sequencing may be used to help confirm whether an intronic variant identified by DNA sequencing predicted to alter mRNA splicing does indeed alter splicing, or to help identify high-priority genes for analysis based on expression differences. A major limitation of RNA sequencing is that expression of some genes is tissue-specific, and thus a gene of interest may not be expressed in an easily accessible tissue, such as a neuron-specific gene not expressed in fibroblasts or WBCs. Furthermore, analysis of RNA sequencing data can be challenging and is not standardized, thus interpretation may vary among clinical laboratories.

LRS and OGM are both only available on a research basis today, although we expect that they will be clinically available in the near future. OGM technology is able to identify structural changes, such as deletions, duplications, or inversions, that may be difficult to identify or characterize with ES or srGS.[34] LRS is typically defined as generating reads longer than 1,000 bp, and has several advantages over traditional short-read based approaches. Similar to OGM, LRS can be used to identify structural differences difficult to detect with conventional testing.[35,36] Two LRS technologies are predominantly used today, one by Pacific Biosciences (PacBio), and the other by Oxford Nanopore Technologies (ONT).[37] While PacBio data are typically of much higher quality than ONT data, ONT data can be generated much more quickly and is cheaper. Recent work on ultra-rapid sequencing has been based on ONT technology and has demonstrated that the technology can be used to sequence critically ill individuals in under 12 hours or to rapidly assess genetic risk in newborns.[38,39] Challenges with LRS include higher cost than conventional approaches and challenges with filtering and prioritizing structural variants for further analysis.

SUMMARY

The introduction of ES led to a dramatic change in our approach to clinical genetic testing. While every genetic modality is clinically useful when appropriately targeted, there are important limitations for each that may warrant further testing or counseling. Overall, individuals and their families today have a higher likelihood of obtaining a precise genetic diagnosis than even a decade ago. There are numerous benefits from improved prognostic information, more accurate counseling, and the ability to benefit from individualized therapies. The future of clinical genetic testing is even more promising, with several new technologies entering the clinical space or being evaluated for clinical use. These new technologies are likely to increase the overall diagnostic rate and simplify clinical genetic testing, leading to improved outcomes for our patients and families.

CLINICS CARE POINTS

- Prior to ordering genetic testing families should be counseled on the possible results, including variants of uncertain significance (VUSs).
- Abnormal genetic testing results should be interpreted in the context of the individual's phenotype, as clinical labs operate with a limited perspective on an individual's phenotype.

- Chromosomal approaches to testing, such as karyotype and SNP array, do not provide information about the sequence of genetic material, and the different types of analyses often have mutually exclusive roles.
- Guidelines, clinical utility, and genetic testing technologies continue to advance rapidly. Current evidence-based guidelines recommend exome sequencing for most children with developmental delays and/or multiple congenital anomalies, especially neonates. If exome sequencing is not available, SNP microarray is still often used as a first-tier test.
- If standard genetic workup, including exome sequencing, is nondiagnostic, consider what may have been missed by prior testing, such as repeat expansions or imprinting disorders.
- If an explanatory variant is identified, it is important to review the results, surveillance recommendations, any management changes, clinical resources, and whether additional family members should undergo testing with the individual and their families.

FUNDING

D.E. Miller is supported in part by the National Institutes of Health, United States Grant DP5OD033357.

DISCLOSURES

D.E. Miller is engaged in a research agreement with Oxford Nanopore Technologies (ONT). ONT has paid for D.E. Miller to travel to speak on their behalf. D.E. Miller holds stock options in MyOme.

AUTHOR CONTRIBUTIONS

A.L. Lenahan, A.E. Squire, and D.E. Miller wrote the article.

ACKNOWLEDGMENTS

The authors thank Angela Miller for editorial assistance.

REFERENCES

1. Pollard S, Weymann D, Dunne J, et al. Toward the diagnosis of rare childhood genetic diseases: what do parents value most? Eur J Hum Genet 2021;29(10):1491–501.
2. The NICUSeq Study Group, Krantz ID, Medne L, et al. Effect of whole-genome sequencing on the clinical management of acutely ill infants with suspected genetic disease: a randomized clinical trial. JAMA Pediatr 2021;175(12):1218–26.
3. Scholz T, Blohm ME, Kortüm F, et al. Whole-exome sequencing in critically ill neonates and infants: diagnostic yield and predictability of monogenic diagnosis. Neonatology 2021;118(4):454–61.
4. Richards S, Aziz N, Bale S, et al. Standards and guidelines for the interpretation of sequence variants: a joint consensus recommendation of the American College of Medical Genetics and Genomics and the Association for Molecular Pathology. Genet Med 2015;17(5):405–24.
5. Grace MR, Hardisty E, Dotters-Katz SK, et al. Cell-free DNA screening: complexities and challenges of clinical implementation. Obstet Gynecol Surv 2016;71(8):477–87.
6. Gregg AR, Skotko BG, Benkendorf JL, et al. Noninvasive prenatal screening for fetal aneuploidy, 2016 update: a position statement of the American College of Medical Genetics and Genomics. Genet Med 2016;18(10):1056–65.

7. Kearney L. Molecular cytogenetics. Best Pract Res Clin Haematol 2001;14(3): 645–69.
8. Marzancola MG, Sedighi A, Li PCH. DNA microarray-based diagnostics. Methods Mol Biol 2016;1368:161–78.
9. Benn P. Uniparental disomy: origin, frequency, and clinical significance. Prenat Diagn 2021;41(5):564–72.
10. Waggoner D, Wain KE, Dubuc AM, et al. Yield of additional genetic testing after chromosomal microarray for diagnosis of neurodevelopmental disability and congenital anomalies: a clinical practice resource of the American College of Medical Genetics and Genomics (ACMG). Genet Med 2018;20(10):1105–13.
11. Rehm HL, Alaimo JT, Aradhya S, et al. Genomic sequencing tests generate less uncertainty and higher diagnostic yield compared to multi-gene panel-based tests: Results of over 1.5 million tests. medRxiv 2022. https://doi.org/10.1101/2022.09.21.22279949.
12. Warr A, Robert C, Hume D, et al. Exome sequencing: current and future perspectives. G3 2015;5(8):1543–50.
13. Lowther C, Valkanas E, Giordano JL, et al. Systematic evaluation of genome sequencing as a first-tier diagnostic test for prenatal and pediatric disorders. Cold Spring Harbor Laboratory 2020;2020. https://doi.org/10.1101/2020.08.12.248526. 08.12.248526.
14. Manickam K, McClain MR, Demmer LA, et al. Exome and genome sequencing for pediatric patients with congenital anomalies or intellectual disability: an evidence-based clinical guideline of the American College of Medical Genetics and Genomics (ACMG). Genet Med 2021;23(11):2029–37.
15. Freed AS, Clowes Candadai SV, Sikes MC, et al. The impact of rapid exome sequencing on medical management of critically ill children. J Pediatr 2020; 226:202–12.e1.
16. Farnaes L, Hildreth A, Sweeney NM, et al. Rapid whole-genome sequencing decreases infant morbidity and cost of hospitalization. Npj Genomic Medicine 2018; 3(1):1–8.
17. Kingsmore SF, Cakici JA, Clark MM, et al. A randomized, controlled trial of the analytic and diagnostic performance of singleton and trio, rapid genome and exome sequencing in ill infants. Am J Hum Genet 2019;105(4):719–33.
18. Miller DT, Lee K, Abul-Husn NS, et al. ACMG SF v3.1 list for reporting of secondary findings in clinical exome and genome sequencing: a policy statement of the American College of Medical Genetics and Genomics (ACMG). Genet Med 2022; 24(7):1407–14.
19. LaDuca H, Farwell KD, Vuong H, et al. Exome sequencing covers >98% of mutations identified on targeted next generation sequencing panels. PLoS One 2017;12(2):e0170843.
20. Lionel AC, Costain G, Monfared N, et al. Improved diagnostic yield compared with targeted gene sequencing panels suggests a role for whole-genome sequencing as a first-tier genetic test. Genet Med 2018;20(4):435–43.
21. Eggermann T, Perez de Nanclares G, Maher ER, et al. Imprinting disorders: a group of congenital disorders with overlapping patterns of molecular changes affecting imprinted loci. Clin Epigenetics 2015;7:123.
22. Ellerby LM. Repeat expansion disorders: mechanisms and therapeutics. Neurotherapeutics 2019;16(4):924–7.
23. Barbosa-Gouveia S, Vázquez-Mosquera ME, González-Vioque E, et al. Utility of gene panels for the diagnosis of inborn errors of metabolism in a metabolic reference center. Genes 2021;12(8). https://doi.org/10.3390/genes12081262.

24. Sánchez Fernández I, Loddenkemper T, Gaínza-Lein M, et al. Diagnostic yield of genetic tests in epilepsy: a meta-analysis and cost-effectiveness study. Neurology 2019. https://doi.org/10.1212/WNL.0000000000006850.

25. Kubota T, Sutcliffe JS, Aradhya S, et al. Validation studies of SNRPN methylation as a diagnostic test for Prader-Willi syndrome. Am J Med Genet 1996;66(1): 77–80.

26. Brioude F, Netchine I, Praz F, et al. Mutations of the Imprinted CDKN1C Gene as a cause of the overgrowth beckwith-wiedemann syndrome: clinical spectrum and functional characterization. Hum Mutat 2015;36(9):894–902.

27. Hunter J, Rivero-Arias O, Angelov A, et al. Epidemiology of fragile X syndrome: a systematic review and meta-analysis. Am J Med Genet 2014;164A(7):1648–58.

28. Feldman EA. The genetic information nondiscrimination act (GINA): public policy and medical practice in the age of personalized medicine. J Gen Intern Med 2012;27(6):743–6.

29. Cakici JA, Dimmock DP, Caylor SA, et al. A prospective study of parental percep-tions of rapid whole-genome and -exome sequencing among seriously ill infants. Am J Hum Genet 2020;107(5):953–62.

30. Deignan JL, Chung WK, Kearney HM, et al. Points to consider in the reevaluation and reanalysis of genomic test results: a statement of the American College of Medical Genetics and Genomics (ACMG). Genet Med 2019;21(6):1267–70.

31. Murdock DR, Rosenfeld JA, Lee B. What has the undiagnosed diseases network taught us about the clinical applications of genomic testing? Annu Rev Med 2022; 73:575–85.

32. Glinos DA, Garborcauskas G, Hoffman P, et al. Transcriptome variation in human tissues revealed by long-read sequencing. Nature 2022;608(7922):353–9.

33. Castel SE, Levy-Moonshine A, Mohammadi P, et al. Tools and best practices for data processing in allelic expression analysis. Genome Biol 2015;16:195.

34. Neveling K, Mantere T, Vermeulen S, et al. Next-generation cytogenetics: comprehensive assessment of 52 hematological malignancy genomes by optical genome mapping. Am J Hum Genet 2021;108(8):1423–35.

35. Miller DE, Sulovari A, Wang T, et al. Targeted long-read sequencing identifies missing disease-causing variation. Am J Hum Genet 2021. https://doi.org/10.1016/j.ajhg.2021.06.006.

36. Cohen ASA, Farrow EG, Abdelmoity AT, et al. Genomic answers for children: Dynamic analyses of >1000 pediatric rare disease genomes. Genet Med 2022; 24(6):1336–48.

37. Logsdon GA, Vollger MR, Eichler EE. Long-read human genome sequencing and its applications. Nat Rev Genet 2020;21(10):597–614.

38. Galey M, Reed P, Wenger T, et al. 3-hour genome sequencing and targeted anal-ysis to rapidly assess genetic risk. medRxiv 2022;2022. https://doi.org/10.1101/2022.09.09.22279746.

39. Gorzynski JE, Goenka SD, Shafin K, et al. Ultrarapid nanopore genome sequencing in a critical care setting. N Engl J Med 2022;386(7):700–2.

Supporting Parents Throughout the Genetic Testing Process and New Diagnosis

Pilar L. Magoulas, MS, CGC[a,b,*]

KEYWORDS

- Genetic counseling • Genetic testing • Diagnostic odyssey • New diagnosis
- Genetic syndrome

KEY POINTS

- The genetic diagnostic process and receiving a new diagnosis can cause stress, anxiety, and uncertainty for families.
- This process can be positively and negatively influenced by parent and provider interactions.
- Factors that increase patient satisfaction with this process include being provided up-to-date, balanced information in a compassionate and caring manner and providing parent-to-parent resources.
- The genetics care provider is equipped and trained to address the support and informational needs of the parents to aid in improved coping, adaptation, and adjustment to a new diagnosis.

INTRODUCTION

The realization that your child may have significant medical and/or developmental problems can cause significant stress and anxiety for parents.[1,2] Increased parental stress can be associated with poorer parental psychosocial functioning, coping, and adaptation, which can in turn impact the child's overall health, well-being, and developmental and behavioral outcomes.[3–5] How parental stress is managed in the initial phases of receiving a diagnosis can impact long-term coping and adaption to their child's disability or diagnosis.[6–8] That stress may be exacerbated when the molecular or etiologic diagnosis remains elusive, as it does in a majority of patients who

[a] Texas Children's Hospital, Houston, TX, USA; [b] Department of Molecular and Human Genetics, Baylor College of Medicine, Houston, TX, USA
* Corresponding author. Department of Molecular and Human Genetics, Baylor College of Medicine, 6701 Fannin Street, Suite 1560, Houston, TX 77030
E-mail address: magoulas@bcm.edu

Pediatr Clin N Am 70 (2023) 917–928
https://doi.org/10.1016/j.pcl.2023.05.005
0031-3955/23/© 2023 Elsevier Inc. All rights reserved.

undergo clinical genetic testing. Thus, finding ways to mitigate that stress early on can, in turn, increase parental adaption to their child's medical or developmental concerns and receipt of an underlying diagnosis.

Many studies have demonstrated the importance of having an early and confirmed genetic diagnosis in a child.[2,9] Benefits include tailoring medical management, supervision, and referrals to other subspecialists based on the diagnosis, receiving prognostic information about what to expect developmentally and medically as the child gets older, obtaining access to social support networks and services, and facilitating connections with other parents who have children with similar conditions.[9] However, despite the benefits, receiving a genetic diagnosis can be challenging as the family learns to cope with their new reality. Parents often report the need for emotional support, information about the condition, and connections with other parents both in the immediate aftermath of receiving a diagnosis and in the first year following receipt of a diagnosis.[1,10,11] This can present additional challenges if the underlying genetic condition is very rare, if there is little information about the condition, or if the condition is a newly discovered neurodevelopmental syndrome where information about the clinical features, prognosis, and long-term outcomes are scarce.[12]

How information is disseminated to families and the interactions with the health care provider team can both positively and negatively influence parental coping and adaption during this time. Therefore, awareness of the roles that geneticists, genetic counselors, and other health care providers can play in this process can significantly influence how the parents process and receive this information, thereby hopefully improving their diagnostic experience. Yet parents often express dissatisfaction with how a diagnosis or difficult news is communicated to them.[2,11,13] Factors that have been identified as being related to increased parental satisfaction include having the health care provider show empathy and compassion when giving difficult news, the certainty of the diagnosis, being provided written information on the condition, offering to connect with other parents of children with similar conditions, and outlining steps for further follow-up.[7,10,11,14]

These insights have led to development of frameworks for giving difficult news (such as a genetic diagnosis) to parents, some of which will be highlighted in further detail in the following sections.[10,11] However, clinicians should recognize that the diagnostic process, often called the diagnostic odyssey or journey, begins at the time that there is a suspicion of an underlying medical or developmental concern in the child, not just at the time of disclosure of a diagnosis. Thus, pediatricians and other primary health care providers also play an integral role in this process for families since they may be among the first care providers to recognize a concern in the child that warrants further evaluation, referrals, and/or genetic testing. Providing information and support to parents as they navigate the diagnostic journey from before, during, and after receiving a genetic diagnosis is essential to parental satisfaction and adaption to difficult news. This review will provide guidance and a framework for providing support to parents throughout the genetic diagnostic odyssey, including, but not limited to, the genetic testing process and receipt of a diagnosis by highlighting critical components to consider at different time points.

BEFORE THE GENETIC DIAGNOSIS: RECOGNITION AND REFERRALS

The pediatrician or primary care provider may be one of the first to initially suspect an underlying medical or developmental concern in a child that warrants additional evaluation from specialists. Communication regarding this suspicion should be done in a sensitive and caring manner with appropriate referrals placed to specialists, such as geneticists, for further diagnostic evaluation. However, preparatory information about the reason for referral to genetics and/or the referral process is often lacking.[15] In one study of 20 families who were referred to a genetics clinic for further evaluation of their child, none of the families remembered being given any information about the process of the referral.[15] This uncertainty about the referral process or what the genetics appointment may entail can lead to unrealistic expectations about the nature of the visit, what information may be provided to families, and dissatisfaction with the referral and genetic evaluation process.

Referrers (the pediatrician, primary care provider, or other specialists) should clearly explain the reason that they are referring the child to a genetics specialist (ie, noting specific medical or developmental features), what they may expect from that visit (ie, an evaluation and possible genetic testing to determine the cause of the features), and why it is important (ie, to further understand the condition in the child to help guide treatment and management). Likewise, at the time of receiving the referral, genetics clinics can also provide families with a summary of what to expect during the genetics clinic appointment so that there is a baseline understanding of the process, particularly with regards to the structure of the session, potential genetic testing options, and timing of results. Without having a clear understanding of the genetics referral or evaluation process, families report unnecessary fears and anxieties with regards to what information will be provided about their child.[15]

Initial Genetics Clinic Visit

During the initial genetics visit, contracting, which is the process by which the geneticist or genetic counselor and patient mutually reach agreement about the goals of the session, should be performed to set expectations about the visit.[16] This can include[17]

- Establishing rapport through verbal and nonverbal interaction or through interpreters
- Establishing a mutually agreed-upon genetic counseling agenda with the patient
- Eliciting patient concerns, expectations, and perceptions
- Determining the knowledge base of the patient
- Assessing the patient's ethno-cultural background, traditions, health beliefs, attitudes, lifestyles, and values
- Outlining the genetic evaluation process.

In addition, introducing the providers present during the visit (ie, residents, genetic counselors, nurse practitioners, other learners) and explicitly stating their roles within the process can aid in the understanding of what support and resources they can offer the family. In one study of parents who received a genetic diagnosis, most participants expressed that they did not understand what the role of a genetic counselor was supposed to be, whereas in other studies, there was a significant correlation between positive parental experience and the presence of a genetic counselor.[18,19] Genetic counselors have extensive training in medical genetics and psychosocial counseling. Thus, by explaining the roles of the providers at the initial evaluation, this may allow the parents to become familiar with the services or assistance that they provide, which may ease communication and improve satisfaction with the team throughout the diagnosis process.

Pretest Counseling

Another important component of the genetics clinic visit is pretest counseling that should occur prior to any genetic testing. Pretest counseling should include the components outlined in **Box 1**. In addition, providers should also discuss the yield, or likelihood of obtaining a "positive" or diagnostic result. The diagnostic yield of genetic testing has increased with the advent of clinical exome and genome sequencing;

Box 1
Components of pretest counseling

- The specific genetic test(s) being considered

- Types of results that may be returned (ie, positive, negative, variants of uncertain significance) and what they may indicate

- The possible need for testing other family members to aid in interpretation

- Turnaround time for when results can be expected

- How the results will be disclosed/communicated to family (ie, phone call, in-person visit, electronic health record messaging)

- Consent process including a discussion of medically actionable/incidental/secondary findings

- Cost of the test and insurance coverage

- Logistics of sample collection (blood, buccal, saliva) and shipment

---

however, over half of individuals who get clinical exome sequencing will still not have a recognized genetic etiology.[20] Thus, in addition to consenting regarding the types of results that may return with exome and genome sequencing, specific discussion and consent should be obtained regarding the possibility of future updated results in the event of an initial nondiagnostic test result. Parents may overestimate the likelihood that genetic testing will give them an "answer" to their child's health or developmental problems, even in spite of extensive pretest counseling.[21] Parents have expressed hope and the belief that the referral to genetics was made to provide a diagnosis.[15] Therefore, providing a realistic estimate of the likelihood of getting a genetic diagnosis (now or in the future) should be done at the initial visit and repeated during subsequent encounters so as to mitigate potential disappointment in the absence of a confirmed genetic etiology.

Genetic testing is not limited to being solely performed in genetics clinics. Many non-genetics care providers, such as neurologists, cardiologists, or immunologists, are ordering genetic testing directly from their respective clinics with or without involvement of a genetic counselor or genetics-trained specialist. Therefore, in the absence of referrals to genetics care providers, careful discussion and pretest counseling should be performed so that the family has clear expectations of the genetic testing process and types of results that may be returned.

RECEIVING THE GENETIC DIAGNOSIS: DISCLOSURE OF RESULTS

Receiving a genetic diagnosis can often come as a shock to parents, particularly in the newborn setting or if the parents were not expecting it. In some cases, a genetic diagnosis can be seen as a relief for finally having an answer to a question that they have long sought after. However, how this information is communicated to families can have a lasting impact on their ability to adapt and cope with the diagnosis, while significantly influencing the perception of their experience with their health care team. Parents often vividly recall the emotions evoked when given difficult news or a diagnosis in their child, and overwhelmingly, the experiences are often perceived as negative.[10,11,18]

Giving Difficult News

Guidelines for disclosing difficult news to patients have been proposed for decades, yet there seems to be little improvement in the satisfaction of parents on the receiving end of this news despite the published recommendations.[11,22] Nevertheless, feedback generated from parents who receive a genetic diagnosis or difficult news highlights several important points that the health care team needs to consider when disclosing results (**Table 1**). Result disclosure can occur in person during an outpatient clinic visit, during an inpatient hospitalization, via telephone, or video conferencing (ie, telemedicine). If the diagnosis is given in the inpatient setting, providers should be sensitive to the additional stress and anxiety that parents of hospitalized children may face.[3] Regardless of the actual physical location of where the result disclosure occurs,

Table 1 Components of a result disclosure session	
Setting	• Have ample seating for everyone present. Standing may give the impression that the provider does not have time or is in a rush • Identify a quiet, private location • Minimize distractions (ie, cell phones, pagers) and physical barriers (such as desks and tables) between the parents and providers • Have both parents present if possible

Information giving	• Review test(s) that were ordered and results
	• Provide verbal and up-to-date written information regarding the diagnosis including:
	  ○ Genetic cause and inheritance (recurrence risk can be discussed at a later date pending parental discretion and/or family-planning)
	  ○ Prognosis
	  ○ Management/treatment options
	  ○ Consensus or management guidelines (if available)
	• Focus on abilities and what the child can and will be able to do, not just disabilities or anticipated medical/developmental problems that may occur
	  * Note that parents may vary in the amount of information they want at the initial disclosure session, so this should be tailored to their individual needs.

Language	• Limit the use of medical terminology and jargon; use simple terminology • Use child's name • Use person first language (ie, "Children with Down syndrome" rather than "Down's children.") • Show warmth, compassion, and empathy • Do not rush the disclosure—take time and pause for questions and understanding
Support and resources	• Provide support group information (if available) • If newly described syndrome/very rare, review social media sites or encourage parents to connect with support groups related to a pertinent feature within the syndrome (ie, epilepsy, heart defect, brain malformation, autism) or local parent-to-parent organizations. • Offer connections with other parents • Review research options or clinical trials (if available)
Next steps	• Outline the next steps and follow-up plan (ie, referrals, recommendations, additional tests, imaging, etc.) • Provide resources on services that may be available (ie, early childhood intervention, disability services, educational planning) • Summarize the information provided and solicit additional questions or provide clarification • Offer to follow up via phone or electronic communication within 1–2 weeks for informal check-in with the family.

the components of a result disclosure session should remain relatively consistent across all settings.

Psychosocial Needs of Parents

Recognizing and addressing the psychosocial needs of parents who receive a genetic diagnosis is crucial to improving their diagnostic experience and overall long-term coping and adaption. In one study that solicited parents' reactions to receiving a genetic diagnosis, only a few parents surveyed said that they had received adequate emotional support during the diagnostic session.[18] Acknowledgment and validation of the types of emotions that parents may feel when receiving this information should be performed throughout the diagnostic process, not just at the time of result disclosure. Some common reactions and feelings that may occur include shock, relief, and varying stages of grief such as denial, anger, sadness, bargaining, and eventually, acceptance.[10,12] It is important to note that parents may go through these stages at different times, in a nonlinear fashion, or to varying degrees, even within the same family. Therefore, giving the parents the time and space to express these emotions, validate their feelings, and provide support and guidance as they navigate this process can improve their experience. There may be times when the clinician suspects that one or both parents may benefit from formal counseling or therapy outside of the genetics clinic. If so, then referrals to counselors or therapists may be indicated.

Factors that have been shown to relate to a more positive diagnostic experience include when the genetics team is less verbally dominant (ie, parents feel like active members of the conversation and not just passive receivers of information), when sufficient emotional support and counseling are provided, when medical jargon and terminology is limited or simplified, when positive aspects of the condition are discussed, and a sense of hope is provided.[11,18] In addition, parents may feel powerless and desire a sense of control when faced with a situation that is outside of their control, such as having a child with a genetic condition.[2] Thus, they may seek tasks or actions to regain a sense of control, such as gathering information, connecting with other families, or researching treatment or management options. By taking a more active role in their child's needs, parents may increase their confidence in their abilities to care for their child and create new images of what their and their child's futures may look like.[2] Genetic counselors and geneticists are specifically trained to guide parents throughout the process by providing hope while acknowledging the grief and emotional fluctuations that can occur.

AFTER THE DIAGNOSIS: ADAPTING AND ADJUSTING

Once the child has received a genetic diagnosis, this may be the end of the diagnostic odyssey for the clinician, but the beginning of an entirely new journey for the family. Thus, the care and support that they receive in the immediate aftermath of receiving the diagnosis and in subsequent encounters can be just as crucial to the coping and adaptation process as in the initial disclosure session. The role of the genetics care provider in the care of the child with a genetic condition should not end once a diagnosis is made, but rather develop and evolve with the changing needs of the family. As the family settles into the diagnosis and their new reality, the genetics care provider is in a unique role as a specialist who can look holistically at the child and serve as their advocate by assessing their needs and those of the family over time.

As outlined previously, parents may experience a myriad of reactions to receiving a genetic diagnosis. During the disclosure session, the amount of information provided to parents may be welcome to some but overwhelming to others. It may take time for parents to absorb and process the information as it pertains to their child, their health, and their future. Therefore, awareness of this next phase as parents transition from seeking a diagnosis to now caring for a child with a genetic condition is warranted.

In one study that assessed the support needs of parents caring for a child with intellectual disability in the first year of life, three main themes were identified. These included (1) emotional support as they adjusted to this new role; (2) informational support and a quest for knowledge; and (3) peer-to-peer support and connections with other parents.[1] Providers should offer a follow-up appointment a few months after the initial disclosure session to review the diagnosis again, assess their social support structure, clarify any uncertainties or questions, and provide emotional and psychosocial support as needed. Parents have stated that they specifically want more information that presents a more positive or hopeful view of their child and diagnosis.[1,11] Syndrome-specific support groups; genetics organizations, such as Global Genes (http://globalgenes.org), National Organization for Rare Disorders (http://www.raredisease.org), and Genetic Alliance (http://geneticalliance.org); and social media syndrome groups, among others, can be helpful resources that provide this information while facilitating connection with other parents. The benefits of connecting with other parents cannot be overstated for it has consistently been recognized by parents as something they desire that is beneficial to their adaptation. It can improve parental well-being by providing emotional support, receiving helpful advice, and alleviating feelings of isolation.[1,6,9–12]

In addition, parents may need practical information with regards to disability, education, and therapeutic services that may be available to their children. These services can vary by country, state, and school districts, so connecting parents with local social services or parent-to-parent groups who have navigated these services can be beneficial.

Children with genetic conditions may have complex care needs that require the help of many different specialists. The genetics care provider can help facilitate communication between specialists to help the families navigate their growing health care team. By providing practical tips, such as having a medical binder organized by specialty, the parents can take additional steps in playing an active role in their child's health care needs.

Once parents have adjusted to the diagnosis, they may be open to seek other opportunities that may benefit their child, such as participating in research studies or clinical trials and learning about new treatment or developments. The genetics care provider can help facilitate these discussions with the family and other experts in the field. In addition, as the child continues to age, the providers can discuss and assist parents in new transitions such as those that pertain to the adult health care and adult developmental services systems.

While most of the emphasis has been on how parents cope and adapt to a new diagnosis in their child, the effects and impact on other family members can be significant. Awareness by the genetics care provider of how the genetic diagnostic experience and receipt of a new diagnosis can impact siblings, grandparents, and other family members should be acknowledged and addressed. Syndrome-specific resources, other types of written materials, such as children's books or disorder guides, and social support resources exist for siblings and grandparents of children who have a genetic condition. Including the entire family in this process and directly assessing their needs may assist in the adjusting to the new diagnosis.

NONDIAGNOSTIC GENETIC TESTING

It is important to consider that a majority of the patients that receive genetic testing may not receive a genetic diagnosis despite a clinical suspicion for an underlying genetic etiology.[20] This will inevitably present additional challenges and uncertainties for both the clinician and the family. Parents have stated that they prefer certainty in the diagnosis for this allows them to gather information, connect with other parents, and start the path toward coping and acceptance once the diagnosis is known.[2] That process can be compromised if, despite extensive genetic testing, a genetic etiology for the child's health and/or developmental concerns is not identified.

In one study that assessed the parental responses to nondiagnostic exome sequencing, parents reported initial disappointment, frustration, and fear yet eventually moved toward acceptance and satisfaction.[21] Interestingly, they all created meaning to explain the lack of a diagnostic result. Thus, even with nondiagnostic results, parents will aim to find a sense of control and meaning regardless of the genetic testing outcome. These findings and emotional reactions were mirrored in parents who received a diagnosis, but the diagnosis was a newly described genetic condition with limited individuals reported in the literature.[12] These parents overwhelmingly expressed uncertainty about their child's health and future, despite having a diagnosis, and sought to connect with other families, thus reinforcing an underlying theme for parents of children with suspected genetic conditions of wanting connections with other parents.

Genetics care providers should be cognizant about the potential effects and emotional implications that having a nondiagnostic result may have for a family, particularly for those who have extensively searched for an answer. Families can be referred to research studies for undiagnosed individuals or to support groups for families who do not have a diagnosis, such as the SWAN (Syndromes Without A Name) organizations that have branches in different countries.

ETHNOCULTURAL SENSITIVITY

All the studies described here evaluated parental reactions to receiving a genetic diagnosis and the psychosocial and emotional needs in parents or caregivers who were English-speaking. Without having data on the experience, emotional, coping, and support needs of parents who speak other languages, we are left to extrapolate and generalize information to other cultures, ethnicities, and ancestries who may not speak English fluently. This is a disservice to these families whose needs may or may not be similar to those of primarily English-speaking families.

This barrier can present challenges at each of the aforementioned steps—the referral process, pretesting counseling, result disclosure, and follow-up after receiving a diagnosis. The use of medical interpreters in the clinic setting can assist in this process. Providing the interpreter with an expectation of what the session(s) will entail and the nature of the discussion ahead of time will better enable the interpreter to communicate effectively with patients who need these services.[17] While many syndrome-specific support groups have created written materials in other languages, it can be very difficult to find adequate information to give families. In addition, connecting families with other parents who speak their preferred language can be a challenge. Therefore, the genetics care providers can initiate contact with support organizations or collate their own list of patients of diverse backgrounds who have expressed interest in connecting with other families. Additional research is needed to ascertain the needs and experiences of parents from various cultures, ethnicities, and ancestries. Having a better understanding of these experiences will better enable us to tailor our counseling to families in a culturally sensitive manner.

DISCUSSION

Supporting families throughout the genetic testing process and receiving a genetic diagnosis is a dynamic process between provider and parents that begins as soon as there is a concern in the child that warrants a genetics referral and continues long after the diagnosis has been made. The key components to consider throughout this process as have been outlined throughout this review are illustrated in **Fig. 1**. The components are set within the framework of both families and providers, demonstrating their cyclical relationship. The relationship between the genetics care provider and families will ebb and flow with time and evolve with the changing needs of the family. As has been previously discussed, the emotional reaction of the parents is largely influenced by the diagnostic process.[2] Yet historically, parents have been dissatisfied with how a diagnosis or difficult news has been communicated to them.[11] The interaction between families and genetics care providers can have a significant impact on long-term parental coping and adaptation.[6,7,18] Thus, genetics care providers are particularly attuned to provide support to parents throughout the genetic diagnostic process in a way that facilitates successful coping, adaption, and increased parental satisfaction.

Before genetic testing is initiated, setting expectations about what the family can expect during the genetics clinic visit can readjust pre-existing expectations and improve parental satisfaction while allaying fears and anxieties that they may have had prior to the visit. The time between being referred for a genetics evaluation and getting a genetic diagnosis can take years. Yet there is increasing evidence that parental satisfaction is improved when there is a reduced time between suspicion of a diagnosis and getting a diagnosis.[23,24] In a large study that assessed the experience of parents of children with Down syndrome, nearly all parents wished that they had been informed earlier, as soon as their physician suspected the diagnosis.[11] However, parents who have had a longer diagnostic odyssey have also reported less negative experiences than those with shorter ones, which was attributed to their readiness to receive a diagnosis and acceptance of their child's health or developmental concerns even before receiving a diagnosis.[18] Providing clear expectations about the

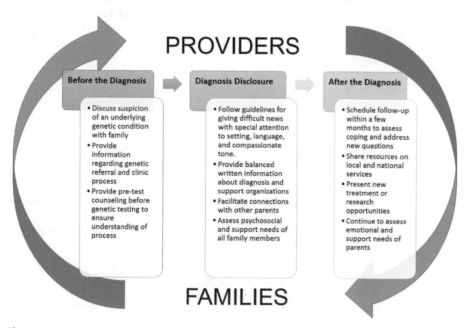

Fig. 1. Recommendations for supporting parents throughout the genetic testing process within the dynamic interaction between care providers and parents.

genetic testing and diagnostic process to families can minimize frustrations that may occur when waiting for genetic testing.

Giving a genetic diagnosis requires a special skill set that should take into account the setting, language used, provider empathy, dissemination of balanced information, and facilitation of parent-to-parent connections. The value of the diagnosis to parents can be unique to each family. In one study that assessed parents' perceived value of a diagnosis for intellectual disability, validation was the most common reason for parents to want a diagnosis [9]. Receiving validation and confirmation of a cause for their child's developmental or cognitive impairments provided them with the confidence to obtain necessary and relevant information to be able to advocate for their child.

After a diagnosis is received, recognition from the health care providers that there is no one right way to cope or adapt to receiving a diagnosis in a child is essential. Displaying compassion and empathy while providing relevant and pertinent information to families as they embark on this new journey can impact parents' overall diagnostic experience. Receiving a diagnosis is like closing one chapter whose focus was on finding an answer to a question that parents may have been seeking for years, but it opens up an entirely new chapter that will extend into the life of their child and family. This new chapter may present more questions that may not have answers, which can be frustrating for parents who seek certainty in the face of uncertainty and action when feeling powerless. As care providers, we need to recognize this transitional period, solicit feedback from parents, and provide adequate support based on their individual needs.

SUMMARY

Receiving a diagnosis is a life-changing event for all family members. It is a crucial time where the parents are learning about their child's specific needs and the new diagnosis, while trying to process, adjust, and cope as they create new images for a future redefined. They are building their confidence in their abilities as parents to care for a child with a genetic condition. There may be fear and uncertainty as they navigate this new territory, and thus, having providers who are able to provide hope and ongoing emotional and informational support before, during, and after receiving a diagnosis can help ease this transition and positively impact the parental diagnostic experience.

CLINICS CARE POINTS

- Receiving a genetic diagnosis can be challenging for individuals and family members.
- Families experience a range of emotions as they learn to cope with the diagnosis.
- Genetics providers are equipped to address the medical, educational, and psychosocial needs of families throughout the genetic testing process and receiving a diagnosis.

DISCLOSURES

The author has no commercial or financial conflicts of interest to disclose.

REFERENCES

1. Douglas T, Redley B, Ottmann G. The first year: The support needs of parents caring for a child with an intellectual disability. J Adv Nurs 2016;72(11):2738–49.

2. Graungaard A, Skov L. Why do we need a diagnosis? A qualitative study of parents' experiences, coping and needs, when the newborn child is severely disabled. Child Care Health Dev 2007;33(3):296–307.
3. Commodari EJ. Children staying in hospital: A research on psychological stress of caregivers. Ital J Pediatr 2010;36(1):40.
4. Mitchell S, Hilliard M, Mednick L, et al. Stress among fathers of young children with type 1 diabetes. Fam Syst Health 2009;27(4):314–24.
5. Cummings ME, Keller PS, Davies PT. Towards a family process model of maternal and paternal depressive symptoms: Exploring multiple relations with child and family functioning. JCPP (J Child Psychol Psychiatry) 2005;46:479–89.
6. Taanila A, Syrjälä L, Kokkonen J, et al. Coping of parents with physically and/or intellectually disabled children. Child Care Health Dev 2002;8(1):73–86.
7. Davies R, Davis B, Sibert J. Parents' stories of sensitive and insensitive care by pediatricans in the time leading up to and including diagnostic disclosure of a life-limiting condition in their child. Child Care Health Dev 2003;29:77–83.
8. Karasavvidis S, Avgerinou C, Lianou E, et al. Mental retardation and parenting stress. Int J Caring Sci 2011;4(1):21–31.
9. Makela N, Birch P, Friedman J, et al. Parental perceived value of a diagnosis for intellectual disability (ID): A qualitative comparison of families with and without a diagnosis for their child's ID. Am J Med Genet 2009;149(11):2393–402.
10. Dent KM, Carey JC. Breaking difficult news in a newborn setting: Down syndrome as a paradigm. Am J Med Genet C 2006;142C(3):173–9.
11. Skotko B. Mothers of children with Down syndrome reflect on their postnatal support. Pediatrics 2005;115(1):64–77.
12. Inglese C, Elliott A, CAUSES Study, Lehman A. New developmental syndromes: Understanding the family experience. J Genet Counsel 2019;28(2):202–12.
13. Pearson P, Simms K, Ainsworth C, et al. Disclosing special needs to parents. Have we got it right yet? Child Care Health Dev 1999;25:3–14.
14. Quine L, Rutter D. First diagnosis of severe mental and physical disability: A study of doctor-parent communication. JCPP (J Child Psychol Psychiatry) 1994;35:1273–87.
15. Skirton H. Parental experience of a pediatric genetic referral. MCN Am J Matern/Child Nurs 2006;31(3):178–84.
16. McCarthy Veach P, LeRoy BS, Callanan NP. Structuring genetic counseling sessions: initiating, contracting, ending, and referral. In: Facilitating the genetic counseling process. Cham (Switzerland): Springer; 2018. p. 93–121. https://doi.org/10.1007/978-3-319-74799-6_6.
17. Hampel H, Grubs RE, Walton CS, et al, American Board of Genetic Counseling 2008 Practice Analysis Advisory Committee. Genetic counseling practice analysis. J Genet Couns 2009;18(3):205–16.
18. Ashtiani S, Makela N, Carrion P, et al. Parents' experiences of receiving their child's genetic diagnosis: A qualitative study to inform clinical genetics practice. Am J Med Genet 2014;164(6):1496–502.
19. Waxler JL, Cherniske EM, Dieter K, et al. Hearing from parents: the impact of receiving the diagnosis of Williams syndrome in their child. Am J Med Genet 2013;161A(3):534–41.
20. Yang Y, Muzny D, Reid J, et al. linical whole-exome sequencing for the diagnosis of Mendelian disorders. N Engl J Med 2013;369(16):1502–11.
21. Werner-Lin A, Zaspel L, Carlson M, et al. Gratitude, protective buffering, and cognitive dissonance: How families respond to pediatric whole exome

sequencing in the absence of actionable results. Am J Med Genet 2018;176(3): 578–88.

22. Ptacek J, Eberhardt T. Breaking bad news: A review of the literature. JAMA 1996; 276:496–502.

23. Nursey A, Rohde J, Farmer R. Ways of telling new parents about their child and his or her mental handicap: A comparison of doctors' and parents' views. J Ment Defic Res 1991;35:48–57.

24. Baird G, McConachie H, Scrutton D. Parents perceptions of disclosure of the diagnosis of cerebral palsy. Arch Dis Child 2000;83:475–80.

Downstream Assays for Variant Resolution

Epigenetics, RNA Sequnncing, and Metabolomics

Brian J. Shayota, MD, MPH[a,b,*]

KEYWORDS

- Epigenetics • DNA methylation • RNA sequencing • Transcriptomics
- Metabolomics

KEY POINTS

- The increasing utilization of broad-spectrum molecular testing like whole exome and genome testing has led to a growing challenge of interpreting inconclusive results.
- Additional testing methods can provide further evidence in support of or against a particular diagnosis.
- Evaluation of DNA epigenetics, RNA sequencing, and metabolomics are more recent, advanced methods used in variant resolution that have been found to increase the diagnostic yield when used in conjunction with more conventional genetic tests.

INTRODUCTION

Over the past 2 decades, advances in genetic testing methods and the growing availability of such tests to the general population has been met with a shift in how physicians provide personalized medical care to patients. It was only in 2004 that the Human Genome Project first sequenced 99% of the human genome at a cost of nearly $3 billion. Since then, several advances, including next-generation sequencing, have led to a precipitous drop in costs, opening the way for expansive testing methods such as gene panels, whole exome sequencing, and whole genome testing into clinical medicine. However, a foreseeable problem with such testing is that the scientific understanding of those variants in the genetic code that have the potential to cause human disease versus those that have no noticeable monogenic clinical significance remains far from resolved. This problem means that often genetic tests find variants of uncertain significance (VUSs), which may result in additional stress for families

[a] University of Utah, 295 Chipeta Way, Salt Lake City, UT 84108, USA; [b] Primary Children's Hospital, Salt Lake City, UT, USA
* 295 Chipeta Way, Salt Lake City, UT 84108.
E-mail address: brian.shayota@hsc.utah.edu

Pediatr Clin N Am 70 (2023) 929–936
https://doi.org/10.1016/j.pcl.2023.05.006
0031-3955/23/© 2023 Elsevier Inc. All rights reserved.

regarding the uncertainty of a potential genetic diagnosis. Research regarding the impact of inconclusive genetic testing remains scarce, but has, in certain scenarios such as a VUS detected in the *BRCA1/2* genes, shown conflicting evidence, with some studies reporting higher levels of distress following disclosure of uncertain genetic test results.[1-5] This dilemma is also a cause for concern for medical providers, as in when trying to determine the right course of action in regard to costly surveillance and/or surgical intervention in the case of a VUS in *BRCA1/2*. In some scenarios, the expertise of a specialist may be able to rule out or infer a diagnosis even with a VUS, by being able to consider the patient's phenotype with the gene in question or by testing other family members. Unfortunately, this is not often the case, particularly when considering disorders with relatively nonspecific or overlapping presentations.

It is also important to note that despite all the advances made in molecular genetics, there are still limits on the variants that testing laboratories are capable of detecting. Even with comprehensive testing like whole genome sequencing, a genetic diagnosis may be missed for a variety of reasons not limited to poor patient phenotyping to guide the analysis, insufficient gene coverage, missed calls due to laboratory error, and yet-to-be-discovered disease-gene associations.[6] Therefore, genetic test results may not be definitive and follow-up testing may be beneficial.

In an effort to obtain more evidence to either rule in or rule out a diagnosis following inconclusive molecular genetic testing, ancillary testing methods are being increasingly used. Such tests themselves have limitations, but when considered along with other available information, may help to make a genetic diagnosis more definitively. Ancillary tests reviewed in this article help fill the gap in the genomics-to-phenomics pathway, because there are several important steps in between that can be assessed (**Fig. 1**). This article reviews some of the more common ancillary "-omic" tests that are currently clinically available or are in development, such as epigenetic signature (episignature) testing, RNA (ribonucelic acid) sequencing, and metabolomic testing.

Epigenetic Testing

Epigenetics refers to the modification of gene expression not caused by changes in the genetic code itself. This article focuses on DNA methylation, although there are other epigenetic factors like histone modification, noncoding RNAs, and higher-

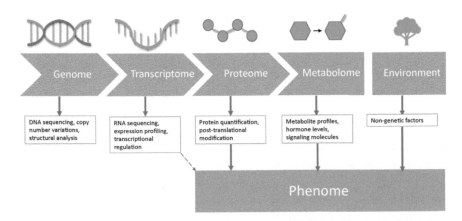

Fig. 1. The pathway by which the genome and various intermediary factors lead to downstream changes that eventually result in a person's unique phenotype.

order chromatin structure factors for which testing methods are less established in clinical medicine. DNA methylation episignatures are defined as the cumulative DNA methylation patterns occurring at multiple CpG dinucleotides across the genome.[7–10] There is a fine balance between DNA methylation, where global loss of methylation has been associated with aging and cancer and gains in global methylation levels have been associated with developmental disorders like trisomy 21.[11–14] Often, targeted methylation testing is only considered for specific pediatric disorders of genomic imprinting such as Prader-Willi syndrome and Angelman syndrome. However, there are several other genetic conditions caused by methylation defects such as Beckwith-Wiedemann syndrome, Russell-Silver syndrome, pseudohypoparathyroidism, Temple syndrome, and Kagami-Ogata syndrome, with likely more that are yet to be discovered. A high index of suspicion is necessary to consider targeted testing for these conditions because they can be missed by more broad tests like chromosome microarrays and exome/genome sequencing, depending on the specific causative defect.

Importantly, it has been shown that genomic DNA methylation patterns can also be influenced by variants in the genetic code itself; this includes genes that encode the methylation machinery like DNA methyltransferases and methyl-CpG-binding proteins, as well as others whose mechanisms are more complex.[10,15] Nonetheless, there is a growing list of Mendelian monogenic disorders that are not caused by the inappropriate inheritance of an imprinted gene but do have a unique episignature pattern. At present, there are as many as 65 genetic syndromes known to have a unique episignature.[16] This fact offers a unique opportunity to assess the relevance of a VUS by obtaining further evidence in support of a diagnosis. The clinical utility of such testing is still being investigated, but in one study, 134 of 136 (98.5%) subjects with a previously identified VUS in a gene known to have a unique episignature received a conclusive test report as being either positive or negative[17]; this has significant clinical impact because even the absence of a methylation signature is considered strong evidence to rule out a condition.

Methylation episignature testing does have some notable limitations at this time. First and foremost, unlike DNA sequencing, DNA methylation is less permanent and can change over time and under the influence of environmental factors.[17] Notably, intraindividual changes over time in DNA methylation levels have been observed and associated with age, creating a type of biological epigenetic clock that can be accelerated by body mass index, nutritional intake, and history of viral infections like human immunodeficiency virus or cytomegalovirus, as well as other factors.[14,18–20] Furthermore, DNA methylation can be altered by certain chemicals and pollutants and can then undergo transgenerational inheritance, whereby abnormal methylation patterns can be seen in future generations.[21–23] Therefore, there still remains a lot to be learned regarding genome-wide methylation patterns and their utility in clinical medicine.

RNA Sequencing

RNA sequencing represents the next step in the central dogma, in which DNA is transcribed to form RNA. As such, if it is unclear what effect a specific DNA variant might have, looking one step further by evaluating the RNA might help resolve this question. RNA sequencing offers the opportunity to identify aberrant transcript events, which include dysregulation of gene expression, abnormal splicing of genes, and monoallelic expression (MAE) of a gene, whereby a single allele is silenced.[24–28] Thus variants that may be missed by whole exome sequencing, such as deep intronic variants causing the skipping and creation of a new exon in *DMD* or the skipping of exon 7 in *SMN1* caused by a variant in a splicing factor binding site, may be found.[28–30] MAE may also be caused by epigenetic factors, like X-chromosome inactivation or imprinting, which may also be missed by some common sequencing tests.[31,32]

RNA sequencing can be done to evaluate a specific gene of interest to follow-up on a VUS, or can be done to look at all ~20,000 genes, referred to as the transcriptome, at once. Transcriptome testing alongside exome sequencing has proven to be a powerful diagnostic tool. The diagnostic yield of transcriptome sequencing has varied between studies depending on the material tested and the selected patient population. For example, patients with a suspected mitochondrial disease and nondiagnostic whole exome sequencing had a diagnostic yield of 10% to 16% when using fibroblasts, whereas patients with undiagnosed muscular disorders had a 35% diagnostic yield when testing a muscle biopsy.[28,33,34] A more generalized approach for patients suspected of any category of genetic disorder enrolled in the Undiagnosed Disease Network found that integration of RNA sequencing along with exome or genome sequencing increased the diagnostic rate from 31% to 38%, and in another similar study, RNA sequencing had a diagnostic rate of 17% after excluding cases solved by whole exome or genome sequencing.[35,36]

One of the current challenges to transcriptomics is determining the optimal tissue for testing because gene expression will vary between different cell types. Although blood is most accessible, there are several genetic conditions caused by variants in tissue-restricted transcripts involving difficult-to-access tissues, like the cerebral cortex or myocardium.[37] The Genotype Tissue Expression (GTEx) project has sought to resolve this by surveying gene expression in multiple human tissues, and the Phenotype-Tissue Expression and Exploration (PTEE) tool was created by Velluva and colleagues[38,39] to guide tissue selection for analysis in different disease contexts. It is also important to note that levels of gene expression can vary with age and certain environmental factors that are yet to be fully understood.[40] Adding even more complexity, a pathogenic variant in a single gene can induce complex changes in the transcriptome including other genes.[41] Nonetheless, the promise of RNA sequencing in clinical medicine continues to grow with each new discovery.

Metabolomics

Untargeted metabolomic testing is an approach to biochemical testing that uses the same concept that favors whole genome testing over gene panels. Rather than picking specific metabolites to investigate, a single metabolomic test can detect over 900 small molecules in a single blood, urine, or cerebrospinal fluid sample.[42,43] More traditional biochemical testing has consisted of specific tests like an acylcarnitine profile, plasma amino acid analysis, and urine organic acid testing. However, these more common biochemical tests are becoming less useful for diagnostic purposes, because many metabolic conditions identified with these techniques have been added to the ever-expanding list of disorders on most newborn screening programs. When comparing the 2 approaches, untargeted metabolomic testing has been found to have a 6-fold higher diagnostic yield than traditional first-tier biochemical testing.[44]

Another advantage of untargeted metabolomic testing is that it does not require a strong index of suspicion for a specific metabolic disorder. This advantage is important because the clinical phenotype for some inborn errors of metabolism can be rather nonspecific. For example, rare disorders of the pentose phosphate pathway can present with nonspecific findings like developmental delay and intellectual disability, but biochemically one would have to consider sending urine polyol testing to make a biochemical diagnosis.[45]

Biochemical testing, regardless of whether it is targeted or untargeted, can also be instrumental in resolving nondiagnostic molecular testing results as well; this may be the case when VUSs are found in genes known to cause metabolic disorders, or when no specific variant is found, but a strong suspicion for a metabolic disorder exists. The metabolome represents one of the final products that contributes directly to the phenome, and most metabolic disorders have a specific metabolic profile that is consistently present.

Biochemical testing, including untargeted metabolomic testing, does come with its own limitations. Similar to episignature and transcriptome testing, there remains a lot to be learned about the metabolome and what changes constitute a genetic disorder and which may be related to other factors like environmental influences or nongenetic illnesses. As such, the interpretation of such testing can be very complex. In addition, unlike the genome, the metabolome is an ever-changing balance of metabolic processes and the profile of some inborn errors of metabolism may only be apparent biochemically when under a sufficient amount of metabolic stress.

SUMMARY

There are several available options for ancillary testing to help with variant resolution. Although most are primarily being used on a research basis, they are becoming increasingly available clinically. This fact is especially true as exome and genome sequencing continues to be more accessible, because these methods have been shown to increase the diagnostic yield when used in conjuncture. Therefore, it will be important for future medical providers to become comfortable with such testing methods in the workup for a suspected genetic disorder.

CLINICS CARE POINTS

- When used in conjuncture with DNA sequencing, ancillary testing to assess for epigenetic signatures, transcriptomics, and metabolomics increases the diagnostic yield.
- Ancillary testing in genetics remains fairly complicated with several additional factors that require consideration when ordering and interpreting results like the type of tissue used and possible environmental influences.

DISCLOSURES

Funding sources: None.

CONFLICTS OF INTEREST

None declared.

REFERENCES

1. Graves KD, Vegella P, Poggi EA, et al. Long-term psychosocial outcomes of BRCA1/BRCA2 testing: differences across affected status and risk-reducing surgery choice. Cancer Epidemiol Biomarkers Prev 2012;21(3):445–55.
2. Dorval M, Gauthier G, Maunsell E, et al. No evidence of false reassurance among women with an inconclusive BRCA1/2 genetic test result. Cancer Epidemiol Biomarkers Prev 2005;14(12):2862–7.

3. van Dijk S, Timmermans DRM, Meijers-Heijboer H, et al. Clinical characteristics affect the impact of an uninformative DNA test result: the course of worry and distress experienced by women who apply for genetic testing for breast cancer. J Clin Oncol 2006;24(22):3672–7.

4. van Dijk S, van Asperen CJ, Jacobi CE, et al. Variants of uncertain clinical significance as a result of BRCA1/2 testing: impact of an ambiguous breast cancer risk message. Genet Test 2004;8(3):235–9.

5. Bramanti SM, Trumello C, Lombardi L, et al. Uncertainty following an inconclusive result from the BRCA1/2 genetic test: A review about psychological outcomes. World J Psychiatry 2021;11(5):189–200.

6. Schobers G, Schieving JH, Yntema HG, et al. Reanalysis of exome negative patients with rare disease: a pragmatic workflow for diagnostic applications. Genome Med 2022;14(1). https://doi.org/10.1186/S13073-022-01069-Z.

7. Aref-Eshghi E, Kerkhof J, Pedro VP, et al. Evaluation of DNA Methylation Episignatures for Diagnosis and Phenotype Correlations in 42 Mendelian Neurodevelopmental Disorders. Am J Hum Genet 2020;106(3):356–70.

8. Aref-Eshghi E, Zhang Y, Liu M, et al. Genome-wide DNA methylation study of hip and knee cartilage reveals embryonic organ and skeletal system morphogenesis as major pathways involved in osteoarthritis. BMC Musculoskelet Disord 2015. https://doi.org/10.1186/s12891-015-0745-5.

9. Yousefi P, Huen K, Davé V, et al. Sex differences in DNA methylation assessed by 450K BeadChip in newborns. BMC Genom 2015;16(1). https://doi.org/10.1186/S12864-015-2034-Y.

10. Robertson KD. DNA methylation and human disease. Nat Rev Genet 2005;6(8):597–610.

11. Jin S, Lee YK, Lim YC, et al. Global DNA hypermethylation in down syndrome placenta. PLoS Genet 2013;9(6). https://doi.org/10.1371/JOURNAL.PGEN.1003515.

12. Wilson AS, Power BE, Molloy PL. DNA hypomethylation and human diseases. Biochim Biophys Acta 2007;1775(1):138–62.

13. Fraga MF, Esteller M. Epigenetics and aging: the targets and the marks. Trends Genet 2007;23(8):413–8.

14. Martin EM, Fry RC. Environmental Influences on the Epigenome: Exposure-Associated DNA Methylation in Human Populations. Annu Rev Public Health 2018;39:309–33.

15. Velasco G, Francastel C. Genetics meets DNA methylation in rare diseases. Clin Genet 2019;95(2):210–20.

16. Levy MA, McConkey H, Kerkhof J, et al. Novel diagnostic DNA methylation episignatures expand and refine the epigenetic landscapes of Mendelian disorders. HGG Adv 2021;3(1):100075.

17. Sadikovic B, Levy MA, Kerkhof J, et al. Clinical epigenomics: genome-wide DNA methylation analysis for the diagnosis of Mendelian disorders. Genet Med 2021;23(6):1065–74.

18. Jones MJ, Goodman SJ, Kobor MS. DNA methylation and healthy human aging. Aging Cell 2015;14(6):924–32.

19. Garagnani P, Bacalini MG, Pirazzini C, et al. Methylation of ELOVL2 gene as a new epigenetic marker of age. Aging Cell 2012;11(6):1132–4.

20. Oblak L, van der Zaag J, Higgins-Chen AT, et al. A systematic review of biological, social and environmental factors associated with epigenetic clock acceleration. Ageing Res Rev 2021;69. https://doi.org/10.1016/J.ARR.2021.101348.

21. Senut MC, Sen A, Cingolani P, et al. Lead exposure disrupts global DNA methylation in human embryonic stem cells and alters their neuronal differentiation. Toxicol Sci 2014;139(1):142–61.

22. Hanna CW, Bloom MS, Robinson WP, et al. DNA methylation changes in whole blood is associated with exposure to the environmental contaminants, mercury, lead, cadmium and bisphenol A, in women undergoing ovarian stimulation for IVF. Hum Reprod 2012;27(5):1401–10.

23. Sen A, Heredia N, Senut MC, et al. Multigenerational epigenetic inheritance in humans: DNA methylation changes associated with maternal exposure to lead can be transmitted to the grandchildren. Sci Rep 2015;5(1):1–10.

24. Albers CA, Paul DS, Schulze H, et al. Compound inheritance of a low-frequency regulatory SNP and a rare null mutation in exon-junction complex subunit RBM8A causes TAR syndrome. Nat Genet 2012;44(4):435–9.

25. Zhao J, Akinsanmi I, Arafat D, et al. A Burden of Rare Variants Associated with Extremes of Gene Expression in Human Peripheral Blood. Am J Hum Genet 2016;98(2):299–309.

26. Guan J, Yang E, Yang J, et al. Exploiting aberrant mRNA expression in autism for gene discovery and diagnosis. Hum Genet 2016;135(7):797–811.

27. Zeng Y, Wang G, Yang E, et al. Aberrant gene expression in humans. PLoS Genet 2015;11(1). https://doi.org/10.1371/JOURNAL.PGEN.1004942.

28. Kremer LS, Bader DM, Mertes C, et al. Genetic diagnosis of Mendelian disorders via RNA sequencing. Nat Commun 2017;8. https://doi.org/10.1038/NCOMMS15824.

29. Qu YJ, Bai JL, Cao YY, et al. A rare variant (c.863G>T) in exon 7 of SMN1 disrupts mRNA splicing and is responsible for spinal muscular atrophy. Eur J Hum Genet 2016;24(6):864–70.

30. Muntoni F, Torelli S, Ferlini A. Dystrophin and mutations: One gene, several proteins, multiple phenotypes. Lancet Neurol 2003;2(12):731–40.

31. Eckersley-Maslin MA, Spector DL. Random monoallelic expression: regulating gene expression one allele at a time. Trends Genet 2014;30(6):237–44.

32. Reinius B, Sandberg R. Random monoallelic expression of autosomal genes: stochastic transcription and allele-level regulation. Nat Rev Genet 2015;16(11):653–64.

33. Cummings BB, Marshall JL, Tukiainen T, et al. Improving genetic diagnosis in Mendelian disease with transcriptome sequencing. Sci Transl Med 2017;9(386). https://doi.org/10.1126/SCITRANSLMED.AAL5209.

34. Yépez VA, Gusic M, Kopajtich R, et al. Clinical implementation of RNA sequencing for Mendelian disease diagnostics. Genome Med 2022;14(1). https://doi.org/10.1186/S13073-022-01019-9.

35. Lee H, Huang AY, Wang L, et al. Diagnostic utility of transcriptome sequencing for rare Mendelian diseases. Genet Med 2020;22(3):490–9.

36. Murdock DR, Dai H, Burrage LC, et al. Transcriptome-directed analysis for Mendelian disease diagnosis overcomes limitations of conventional genomic testing. J Clin Invest 2021;131(1). https://doi.org/10.1172/JCI141500.

37. Montgomery SB, Bernstein JA, Wheeler MT. Toward transcriptomics as a primary tool for rare disease investigation. Cold Spring Harb Mol Case Stud 2022;8(2). https://doi.org/10.1101/MCS.A006198.

38. Lonsdale J, Thomas J, Salvatore M, et al. The Genotype-Tissue Expression (GTEx) project. Nat Genet 2013;45(6):580–5.

39. Velluva A, Radtke M, Horn S, et al. Phenotype-tissue expression and exploration (PTEE) resource facilitates the choice of tissue for RNA-seq-based clinical

genetics studies. BMC Genom 2021;22(1). https://doi.org/10.1186/S12864-021-08125-9.

40. Viñuela A, Brown AA, Buil A, et al. Age-dependent changes in mean and variance of gene expression across tissues in a twin cohort. Hum Mol Genet 2018; 27(4):732.

41. Koks G, Pfaff AL, Bubb VJ, et al. At the dawn of the transcriptomic medicine. Exp Biol Med (Maywood) 2021;246(3):286–92.

42. Kennedy AD, Pappan KL, Donti TR, et al. Elucidation of the complex metabolic profile of cerebrospinal fluid using an untargeted biochemical profiling assay. Mol Genet Metab 2017;121(2):83–90.

43. Kennedy AD, Miller MJ, Beebe K, et al. Metabolomic Profiling of Human Urine as a Screen for Multiple Inborn Errors of Metabolism. Genet Test Mol Biomarkers 2016;20(9):485–95.

44. Liu N, Xiao J, Gijavanekar C, et al. Comparison of Untargeted Metabolomic Profiling vs Traditional Metabolic Screening to Identify Inborn Errors of Metabolism. JAMA Netw Open 2021;4(7). https://doi.org/10.1001/JAMANETWORKOPEN.2021.14155.

45. Shayota BJ, Donti TR, Xiao J, et al. Untargeted metabolomics as an unbiased approach to the diagnosis of inborn errors of metabolism of the non-oxidative branch of the pentose phosphate pathway. Mol Genet Metab 2020;131(1–2): 147–54.

Shedding New Light
Novel Therapies for Common Disorders in Children with Neurofibromatosis Type I

Natasha Pillay-Smiley, DO[a,b,c], Jonathan S. Fletcher, MD, PhD[b,c,d], Peter de Blank, MD[a,b,c], Nancy Ratner, PhD[b,c,*]

KEYWORDS

- MEK inhibitor • Plexiform neurofibroma • Neurofibromatosis type 1
- Low-grade glioma

KEY POINTS

- Neurofibromatosis type 1 is one of a number of inherited disorders, called RASopathies, that result in activation of the RAS-MAPK intracellular signaling pathway.
- The NF1 protein, neurofibromin, is an off signal for RAS-GTPases. When mutated, loss of NF1 function can cause tumors, cognitive dysfunction, and other manifestations.
- Blockade of RAS-MAPK signaling shrinks tumors in most individuals with plexiform neurofibromas and may improve manifestations in related RASopathies.
- MEK inhibitors have proven efficacy in the treatment of NF1-associated tumors, including low-grade gliomas and plexiform neurofibromas.
- Animal models of NF1 are being used preclinically to identify agents that synergize with or augment the effects of MEK inhibition, with the immediate goal of more durable and deeper tumor regressions, for clinical translation.

INTRODUCTION/HISTORY/DEFINITIONS/BACKGROUND

Neurofibromatosis type I (NF1; MIM#162200) is a common, autosomal-dominant inherited disorder predisposing affected individuals to variety of clinical manifestations. The incidence of NF1 is approximately 1 in 3000 live births, occurring at similar rates in

[a] University of Cincinnati College of Medicine, Cincinnati, OH 45229, USA; [b] Division of Experimental Hematology and Cancer Biology, Cancer and Blood Diseases Institute, Cincinnati Children's Hospital Medical Center, 3333 Burnet Avenue, Cincinnati, OH 45229-0731, USA; [c] Cancer and Blood Diseases Institute, The Cure Starts Now Foundation Brain Tumor Center, Cincinnati Children's Hospital Medical Center, Cincinnati, OH 45229, USA; [d] Current Address: Division of Hematology-Oncology, University of Texas Southwestern, Dallas, TX, USA
* Corresponding author. Division of Experimental Hematology and Cancer Biology, Cancer and Blood Diseases Institute, Cincinnati Children's Hospital Medical Center, 3333 Burnet Avenue, Cincinnati, OH 45229-0731.
E-mail address: Nancy.Ratner@cchmc.org

Pediatr Clin N Am 70 (2023) 937–950
https://doi.org/10.1016/j.pcl.2023.05.007
0031-3955/23/© 2023 Elsevier Inc. All rights reserved.

both sexes and across races.[1] In the 1990s, the single NF1 gene, *NF1*, and its protein product, neurofibromin, were discovered. Identification of the causative disease gene and advances in genomics technology now allow for the verification of NF1 diagnoses, identification of rare genotype-phenotype correlations between specific *NF1* pathogenic variants and associated clinical manifestations of disease, and additional evidence that variants in modifier genes contribute to variable disease expressivity. Notably, NF1 is one of a set of disorders called RASopathies, in which individuals have germline mutations in genes in the intracellular RAS–mitogen activated protein kinase (MAPK) pathway. Indeed, work in animal models and clinical trials led to Food and Drug Administration (FDA) approval for use of MEK inhibitors for inoperable plexiform neurofibroma (PN) in NF1; these inhibitors are being tested in other NF1 indications and other RASopathies (see later).

WORLD-WIDE INCIDENCE, DIAGNOSTIC CRITERIA, AND TUMOR MANIFESTATIONS

More than 95% of individuals with NF1 can be diagnosed using National Institutes of Health diagnostic criteria for NF1 defined in 1987; a 2021 consensus group updated these diagnostic criteria. The most important change included evaluation of individuals with no familial history of NF1 by genetic testing.[2,3] Under the revised criteria, a diagnosis of NF1 is made if two or more of the following are present in those without a positive family history of NF1: (1) six or more café-au-lait macules greater than 5 mm in greatest diameter (prepubertal) or greater than 15 mm in greatest diameter (postpubertal); (2) two or more neurofibromas of any type or one PN; (3) axillary or inguinal freckling; (4) optic glioma; (5) in the eye, two or more Lisch nodules in iris, or choroidal bright spots observable by *optical coherence tomography* or *near infrared* imaging; (6) distinctive bone lesions, such as sphenoid bone dysplasia, anterior bowing of the tibia, or pseudoarthrosis of a long bone; and (7) a first-degree relative meeting these criteria, or a heterozygous pathogenic *NF1* gene variant with a variant allele frequency of 50% in apparently normal tissue. Other manifestations of NF1 are common, although not included in the diagnostic criteria; half of individuals with NF1 show motor dysfunction and/or cognitive disfunction, resulting in decreased school performance.[4] Macrocephaly and vascular changes are also common.[5]

A key feature of NF1 is variability in disease manifestations among members of a family, all of whom share a pathogenic *NF1* variant. Twin studies, studies of more distant family members, and sequencing of genomic DNA from individuals with NF1 all suggest that modifier genes contribute to this variability. For example, tumor numbers and numbers of café-au-lait macules are more similar between nearer relatives than more distant relatives.[6]

In affected families, NF1 follows a pattern of autosomal-dominant inheritance. De novo mutations account for half of patients with NF1, highlighting the mutability of the *NF1* gene. Missense, nonsense, splice site alleles, and deletions occur throughout the *NF1* sequence, and are largely loss of function alleles and are generally not recurrent.[7] Pathogenic variants occur throughout the huge *NF1* gene. Few *NF1* gene-related genotype-phenotype relationships have been defined. Indeed genotype-phenotype correlations affect, at most, 5% to 10% of NF1 families; of these, the most common are whole gene deletions, which predispose to more severe cognitive dysfunction and increased tumor burden as compared with most NF1 pathogenic variants.[8]

Some NF1-associated manifestations (eg, cognitive dysfunction) are not known to involve dysregulated cell growth, and cells in the brain may show the *NF1* ± phenotype characteristic of all cells in the body of individuals with NF1. However, many NF1manifestations are hyperplastic or benign neoplastic processes. Cells isolated from these growths, from hyperpigmented spots to tumors, consistently show mutation/loss of both copies of *NF1*, consistent with a tumor suppressor gene function for *NF1*. Examples of tumors showing biallelic variants in the *NF1* gene are neurofibromas and optic pathway glioma (OPG). Cutaneous and subcutaneous (dermal) neurofibromas are superficial, benign nerve tumors that may occur as solitary lesions in normal individuals; multiple dermal neurofibromas often develop in patients with NF1 during puberty, and do not progress to malignancy. Recent study shows that dermal neurofibromas are associated with Schwann cells in nerves that innervate skin appendages.[9] Dermal neurofibromas contain Schwann cells with biallelic *NF1* mutations,[10] and no other known genomic alterations. NF1-associated low-grade glioma typically demonstrate biallelic loss of *NF1* and do not show the *BRAF* aberrations commonly seen in sporadic low-grade glioma.[11-13] Most NF1-associated low-grade glioma show only biallelic variants in the *NF1* gene, although *FGFR1* and *ATRX* alterations may occasionally be present. Similar to low-grade glioma and dermal neurofibromas, PNs, benign tumors that manifest in early life and grow most rapidly in the first decade of life,[14] are associated with biallelic *NF1* loss in tumor Schwann cells.[15] No other recurrent variants are found in these tumors. PNs are disfiguring, and their growth may compress other vital structures, causing significant morbidity.

Individuals with NF1 are also at increased risk of developing aggressive malignant peripheral nerve sheath tumors (MPNST) within a PN; the only cure for MPNST is total surgical resection, which is often not medically feasible given location of nerve-integrated tumor. Unlike NF1-associated gliomas and PN, MPNST carry multiple variants in addition to biallelic *NF1* pathogenic variants. The pathogenesis of MPNST is thought to start with loss of the normal *NF1* allele in Schwann cells followed by loss of additional tumor suppressor genes including *CDKN2A* and then *SUZ12* or EED, after which MPNST are characterized by loss of histone H3 lysine 27 trimethylation.[16,17]

LIFE EXPECTANCY AND PREDISPOSITION TO MALIGNANCY

The overall life expectancy in patients with NF1 is 8 to 20 years less than that of the general population. This is primarily because of early death resulting from disease-associated neoplasia in individuals less than 50 years of age; MPNST is the most common cause of early mortality in adult patients with NF1.[18] Strikingly, the lifetime risk of developing MPNST is estimated at approximately 5% to 10% for the NF1 population, relative to an approximately 0.001% lifetime risk in the general population. In younger patients with NF1, OPG is a major cause of loss of vision and morbidity but rarely early mortality. In addition, individuals with NF1 have a moderately increased (two- to four-fold) risk of a developing malignancies including rhabdomyosarcoma, pheochromocytoma, grade II-IV brain tumors, and breast cancer.[16,19] In total, people with NF1 have a 60% lifetime risk of developing cancer.[16] Children with NF1 are also at increased risk of developing acute myeloid leukemia or myelodysplastic syndrome, especially in response to genotoxic chemotherapy for other tumors, suggesting that the myeloid compartment is particularly sensitive to *NF1* loss.

RELATED DISORDERS: THE RASopathies

NF1 is now recognized as part of a larger family of genetic diseases that regulate the Ras signaling, dubbed RASopathies.[20,21] More than seven distinct RASopathies, associated with 14 different genes involved in Ras pathway signaling, have been identified. Diseases affected include NF1, Legius syndrome, Noonan syndrome, Noonan syndrome with multiple lentigines (formerly called LEOPARD syndrome), Costello syndrome, cardiofaciocutaneous syndrome, Noonan-like syndrome, hereditary gingival fibromatosis, and capillary malformation–arteriovenous malformation. Congenital abnormalities, especially cardiac, facial, and neurologic abnormalities, and tumor predisposition are common overlapping phenotypic features of many of these diseases.

RASopathies are associated with germline pathogenic variants in p21 Ras proteins (encoded by *NRAS, KRAS, HRAS, RRAS, MRAS*), their upstream activators (*CBL, SOS1/2*), or downstream targets *MEK1/MEK2*, and with inactivating variants in negative regulators of Ras signaling, such as *NF1*. Variants, including variants in the small G-proteins *RIT1, RRAS, RASA2/TC21*, the *MRAS/PP1CB/SHOC2* complex, and in *LZTR1*, which normally regulates RAS and/or RIT expression, are also associated with RASopathies; thus, all RASopathy proteins upregulate RAS-MAPK pathway signaling. Ras proteins are central regulators of intracellular signaling in response to extracellular stimuli, such as growth factors, cytokines, and GPCR signaling.[22–25] Activation of membrane-associated growth factor receptors by extracellular ligands facilitates the recruitment of proteins with Ras guanine exchange factor (Ras-GEFs), such as SOS1, to intracellular membranes. Ras-GEFs catalyze the exchange of Ras-bound GDP for GTP, converting inactive Ras-GDP to active Ras-GTP, to activate downstream signaling pathways important for cellular growth, proliferation, differentiation, and survival and modulation of the immune system (**Fig. 1**).[26] *SPRED1* also functions in the Ras pathway; SPRED1, the causative protein in the RASopathy Legius syndrome,[27] brings neurofibromin to the membrane to modulate Ras signaling.[28]

NF1 is a large, multiexon gene, transcribed and translated to produce a 2818 amino acid protein, neurofibromin. Using structural biology methods, it was recently found

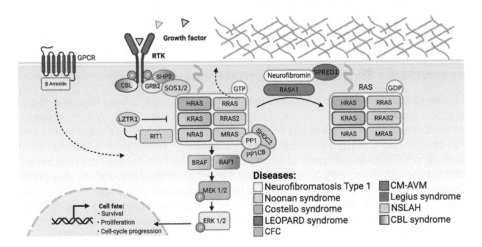

Fig. 1. The RAS-MAPK pathway. In NF1/RASopathies, germline mutation of any of the genes in the Raf/MEK/ERK classical mitogen activated protein kinase (MAPK) pathway results in pathway activation. This can occur through activation of RAS exchange factors (eg, SOS1/2), loss of negative regulators (eg, neurofibromin or RASA1), activating mutations in RAS proteins themselves, or activations of RAS downstream effectors. Mutations in core-pathway interacting proteins, such as SHOC2, LZTR1, and RIT, similarly activate the RAS-MAPK pathway, in which activated Ras-GTP binds Raf (A-RAF, B-RAF, RAF-1) MAPK kinases, inducing Raf dimerization and activation. Activated Raf then phosphorylates MEK (MEK1, MEK2) MAPK kinases. MEK proteins then activate ERK (ERK1, ERK2) MAPKs, amplifying the original signal, and resulting in activating downstream effectors of processes including cellular survival, differentiation, proliferation, and invasion, and inflammatory signaling. CFC, cardiofaciocutaneous; CM-AVM, capillary malformation–arteriovenous malformation.

that neurofibromin exists as a constitutive high affinity dimer in either an "off" or an "on" configuration; in the "on" conformation neurofibromin can interact with RAS-GTP. In this conformation, the neurofibromin GAP-related domain (GRD) negatively regulates Ras by increasing its intrinsic GTPase activity, facilitating the conversion of active RAS-GTP to inactive RAS-GDP.[29,30] Only the neurofibromin dimer in its "on" configuration can interact with Ras.

Missense mutations in *NF1* that selectively reduce the activity of the GRD are sufficient to cause clinical disease, underscoring the functional significance of this domain. Notably, the structural studies of NF1 show that pathogenic variants are most dense in regions encoding the dimerization interfaces and the GRD. Functions have been suggested for other (non-GRD) domains of neurofibromin in regulating its expression, localization, and protein-protein interactions, but their disease relevance remains largely unclear.[31]

MOUSE MODELS OF NEUROFIBROMATOSIS TYPE I

Consistent with the tumor suppressor function of *NF1*, aged mice heterozygous for *Nf1* were predisposed to the development of a variety of malignancies, in which loss of the second copy of *Nf1* was frequently detected.[32,33] However, *Nf1* heterozygous mouse lines did not develop classical features of human disease, such as PN and dermal neurofibromas. The use of Cre-loxP recombinase system to conditionally delete *Nf1* in specific cell populations allowed for the generation of models that are excellent mimics of NF1-associated pathologies.[34] Biallelic deletion of *Nf1* in Schwann cells and Schwann cell precursors in *Dhh*-Cre;*Nf1*[fl/fl] mice was sufficient to induce PN development, and early dermal neurofibromas, demonstrating that an *Nf1* heterozygous background, whereas tumor-promoting, is not a requirement for neurofibroma development.[35] Models of robust dermal neurofibromas have recently been described.[36,37]

Significant immune cell infiltration is present in human and mouse PN,[38] and OPG. Inflammation can act as a driver of neurofibroma development, and precedes tumor development.[39] Given the robust inflammation that characterizes neurofibromas and OPG, investigators have targeted pathways to interfere with the tumor microenvironment. In a 2013 study, Prada and colleagues[38] examined the effects of a CSF1R inhibitor on PN initiation and growth in *Dhh*-Cre;*Nf1*[fl/fl] mice. In established tumors, reduction of tumor growth correlated with macrophage depletion, but, paradoxically, inhibition of CSF1R at 1 month (before tumor formation) enhanced neurofibroma growth in these mice.[38] Like neurofibromas, OPG contain numerous myeloid cells; in mouse and human neurofibromas, these immune cells account for at least a third of all tumor cells.[40]

Mouse and human pharmacologic studies have examined the effects of targeted inhibition of Ras-downstream signaling pathways, in particular, the Raf/MEK/ERK and PI3K/AKT/mTOR pathways. Farnesyltransferase inhibitor showed no effect.[41] Inhibition of mTOR, while reducing tumor burden in mouse models of NF1-associated optic glioma, did not reduce tumor volume in mouse or human PN. Sorafenib, a Raf kinase inhibitor, was not well tolerated in patients.[42,43] In contrast, MEK inhibition is effective in PN, significantly reducing tumor volumes relative to baseline in approximately 70% of mice and then in humans and seemed to have acceptable toxicities.[44–46] Imatinib showed limited efficacy in humans.[47]

CLINICAL IMPLICATIONS OF MEK INHIBITORS IN NEUROFIBROMATOSIS TYPE I

People with NF1 have a 60% lifetime risk of developing cancer,[16] and many individuals with NF1 develop benign tumors. These may be amenable to treatment with MEK inhibitors, because MEK inhibitors are the first FDA-approved pharmacologic treatment of an NF1-associated PN, and their use in other NF1 manifestations is being investigated.

Plexiform Neurofibroma

Of individuals with NF1, 25% to 30% have visible or symptomatic PN and greater than 50% have one or more MRI-detectable PNs.[44,48] The first successful application of MEK inhibitors was documented in NF1-associated PNs based on promising results in mouse models.[45] These lesions can cause significant morbidity based on size, tumor location, and interference with function of the peripheral nerves that the tumors inhabit, including pain, weakness, and loss of function. Given the significant morbidity that can arise from these tumors, a phase 1 study of selumetinib in children with NF1 and inoperable, symptomatic PNs was undertaken. Dombi and colleagues[44] reported the results of this trial and described the side effects of the drug, which were acneiform rash, gastrointestinal effects, and elevation in creatinine kinase. In addition, 71% of children had a partial response (decrease in volume by >20%). A phase II study (SPRINT trial) confirmed a significant partial response in 68% of patients with most having a durable response of more than 1 year.[49] Volume reduction of PN is often variable; although some tumors may reduce significantly in size, others may not be significantly reduced. Correlative studies embedded in the SPRINT trial showed that children had a decrease in pain-intensity scoring and meaningful improvements in quality of life, strength, and mobility.[49] These results have led to FDA and *European Medicines Agency* approval of selumetinib (Koselugo) in the treatment of patients between the ages of 2 and 18 years of age with NF1-associated PN that are inoperative and symptomatic.[48] This was the first FDA approval of a drug for NF1. Responses to MEK inhibitors in PN and OPG are shown in **Fig. 2**.

The effectiveness of other MEK inhibitors in the treatment of PNs are currently being investigated. A study by the NF Clinical Trial Consortium (NF106) showed that the MEK inhibitor mirdametinib had efficacy in children and adults greater than or equal to 16 years old with progressive PNs with a 42% partial response and some reduction in pain.[50] A phase 2 study (NCT03363217) looking at the efficacy of trametinib in

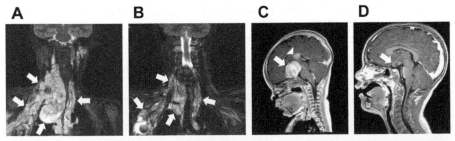

Fig. 2. MRI showing tumors in individuals with NF1 before and after MEK inhibitor treatment. A large cervicothoracic plexiform neurofibroma extending from the skull base to the shoulder girdle shown on MRI using short tau inversion recovery sequence (*A*) before treatment with MEK inhibitor (*arrows*) and (*B*) after more than 5 years of treatment with MEK inhibitor (*arrows*). An enhancing hypothalamic/chiasmatic low-grade glioma (*arrow*) with metastasis (*arrowhead*) projecting from the medial right thalamus is seen in enhanced T1-weighted MRI sequence before MEK inhibitor treatment (*C*) and after 2 years of treatment (*D*). Following treatment, the hypothalamic tumor (*arrow*) is significantly reduced in size and the thalamic lesion has resolved.

patients with NF-1 with PNs or progressive low-grade glioma and a phase II study of binimetinib in children and adults with PNs (NF108-BINI, NCT03231306) are also currently underway. Other targeted agents have also been investigated. Cabozantinib, a multityrosine kinase inhibitor, demonstrated that only 9.5% of PN in pediatric patients had a partial response, although it was more efficacious in a previous trial of adolescents and adults in a phase II (NF105; NCT02101736).[51]

Low-Grade Glioma

OPGs are benign glioma of the optic pathway (optic nerve, chiasm, and tracts), which occur in 5% to 15% of patients with NF1 with a mean age of diagnosis of 5 years. The Pediatric Brain Tumor Consortium conducted a phase 2 study looking at selumetinib in the treatment of children with recurrent, refractory, or progressive low-grade glioma. One of the strata included children with NF1-associated low-grade glioma. In this study, 40% of children had a partial response to selumetinib given orally twice daily, defined as greater than or equal to 50% reduction in bidimensional tumor size, and 60% had stable disease.[52] Similar to PN results, the response of low-grade glioma to MEK inhibition is frequently variable, and regrowth is frequently seen after discontinuation of therapy. With the data from this phase 2 trial, a study was developed and is now underway prospectively comparing selumetinib with a standard of care regimen in previously untreated patients with NF1-associated low-grade glioma (ACNS1831, NCT03871257).

The INSPECT trial (NCT03326388) is examining intermittent dosing schedule of selumetinib in children with progressive or relapsed OPGs or inoperable PN. Tovorafenib, a newer pan-RAF kinase inhibitor, is being used in the LOGGIC/FIREFLY-2 trial in children with progressive low-grade glioma. It is yet to be used in children with NF-1.

Juvenile Myelomonocytic Leukemia

Juvenile myelomonocytic leukemia (JMML) is an aggressive form of childhood leukemia characterized by mutations in the Ras pathway, thus making children with NF1 and other RASopathies at increased risk for this malignancy.[53] JMML presents with a low number of blasts in the peripheral blood or bone marrow because of a lack of maturation arrest during myeloid differentiation, making it challenging to diagnose. It presents mostly in infants and toddlers, and accounts for 1% of all pediatric leukemias. However, the incidence of JMML in children with NF1 is more than 200 times the general population.[54] With preclinical studies demonstrating longer survival and greater disease control in JMML mice models with the use of MEK inhibitors,[55] a pediatric clinical trial using trametinib in relapsed and refractory JMML is now ongoing through the Children's Oncology Group (ADVL1521, NCT03190915). However, results from this trial are not yet available.

Malignant Peripheral Nerve Sheath Tumors

These aggressive sarcomas occur at a median age of 26 to 40 years in patients with NF1 and are often refractory to treatment with a poor overall survival despite surgery, radiation, and chemotherapy.[56] Preclinical models have shown that monotherapy with MEK inhibition is unlikely to be efficacious, and clinical experience has shown that treatment with MEK inhibitor alone does not prevent MPNST. Current clinical trials are investigating combination therapy with MEK inhibitor and other targeted therapies.

Functional Outcomes

Given the impact of NF1-associated tumors on quality of life and morbidity including vision, mobility, pain, and function, clinical trials have used correlative studies to assess patient-reported functional and quality of life outcomes. The Pediatric Brain Tumor Consortium phase 2 study evaluating selumetinib in NF1-associated low-grade gliomas found that 20% of children with OPGs had improvement in visual acuity, whereas 80% remained stable, although this was a small sample of patients with tumors in the optic pathway.[52] The SPRINT trial evaluating selumetinib in children with inoperative PN showed that patients had a decrease in pain-intensity score, and meaningful improvements in quality of life, strength, and mobility.[49] However, treatment with selumetinib did not seem to have a significant effect on scoliosis, bone mineral density, or other bone manifestations of NF1.[57,58] Given these published results, subsequent ongoing clinical trials including ACNS1831, ACNS1833, and the LOGGIC trial have been designed as noninferiority trials to underscore the importance of secondary end points, including patient-reported functional outcomes and assessment of motor, vision, and cognitive function.

Patients with NF1 are at high risk for motor, neurocognitive, and behavioral issues, affecting up to 80% of people with NF1.[4,59–61] Ongoing studies are examining the impact of MEK inhibitor on cognition. A large multicenter cognitive correlative study involving children enrolled on multiple clinical trials for selumetinib in PN revealed that children had clinical improvement on working memory and executive functioning.[61] Similarly, trametinib is being investigated in a phase 2 trial of children with low-grade glioma and PN with neurocognitive assessment as a correlative study.[62] Preliminary results have demonstrated improvement in verbal comprehension and processing speed.[62]

NF1-associated bone dysplasia can also cause significant pain and morbidity. This includes chest wall deformities, idiopathic scoliosis, osteopenia, tibial dysplasia, and pseudoarthrosis.[17,63] Preclinical testing in preclinical models has elucidated the role of MEK inhibitor in bone healing and osteoblast differentiation. A recent study combining MEK inhibitor with a bisphosphonate showed improved BMP2 spine fusion with increased bone density in a murine model.[64] However, a clinical trial of MEK inhibitor with bone morphogenetic protein for children with tibial pseudoarthrosis was unable to recruit sufficient subjects to evaluate this combination.[58]

Side Effects of MEK Inhibitor

As treatment with MEK inhibition becomes more commonplace, identification and surveillance of toxicities has become increasingly important. MEK inhibitors in pediatric patients have been well tolerated overall. The most common side effects noted in clinical trials have been gastrointestinal, including nausea, abdominal pain, weight gain, and diarrhea. In addition, asymptomatic elevation of creatinine kinase and dermatologic toxicity has also been frequently reported. Eczema and acneiform rashes, photosensitivity, lightning of hair color, and paronychia have been seen frequently.[44,52,65] Excellent supportive care measures have been created for mitigation of some of these dermatologic side effects, but 25% to 40% of patients on clinical trials have required dose reduction, or less frequently, discontinuation of therapy.[44,63,65]

Although reported more frequently in adult trials with MEK inhibitors, symptomatic cardiac toxicity has been reported rarely in pediatrics. Asymptomatic decreases in ejection fraction were noted in the low-grade glioma selumetinib trial.[52] Ocular side effects have also been reported in adults ranging from mild to severe. The most common side effects are dry eye, periorbital edema, and retinopathy. More serious side effects include retinal vein occlusion and bilateral retinal detachment. Serious ocular toxicity has not been reported in any of the pediatric MEK inhibitor clinical trials.[44,50,52,65] Routine surveillance for these toxicities, including echocardiograms and ophthalmologic examinations, are recommended while being treated with MEK inhibitors.[63]

THE ROLE OF MEK INHIBITORS IN OTHER RASopathies

Individuals with RASopathies, including Noonan, Costello, and cardiofaciocutaneous,[63,66,67] can develop severe clinical phenotypes, ranging from congenital heart disease, intellectual disability, feeding intolerance, and cancers, such as rhabdomyosarcoma and neuroblastoma.[66,67] No clinical trials exist currently for MEK inhibitors in RASopathies outside of NF1, but preclinical animal model testing shows promising benefit in models of Costello and Noonan syndrome. Recent case reports also describe children with Noonan syndrome treated with trametinib for life-threatening congenital heart disease and lymphatic disorders. Dori and colleagues[68] report significant improvement in a severe protein-losing enteropathy in a child with Noonan syndrome after failing medical and surgical intervention. Similarly, Nakano and colleagues[69] report resolution of chronic chylous effusions in three children. Additional published case studies report reversal of hypertrophic cardiomyopathy.[70,71] However, evidence for the use of MEK inhibitors or other Ras-targeted agents in non-NF1 RASopathies remains in its infancy.

SUMMARY AND FUTURE DIRECTIONS

Despite recent progress in MEK inhibitor treatment of NF1-associated manifestations, much more needs to be done. The development of MEK inhibitor therapy in NF1 has been built on a strong foundation of preclinical investigations, and future directions will rely on further testing in these models. Ongoing preclinical work is needed to identify mechanisms for MEK inhibitor resistance and to help predict the variable effects of MEK inhibitors seen among different patients to identify those who will benefit from this therapy and discover curative treatments. Preclinical models may also help to understand the effect of targeted inhibition on NF1 manifestations that do not seem to require biallelic loss, such as cognitive differences. Furthermore, tumor growth resumes after discontinuation of MEK inhibitor therapy, suggesting that MEK inhibition fails to produce tumor senescence. Rational combinations of MEK inhibition with other therapies (possibly including cytotoxic therapies, immunotherapies, or other targeted agents) are being investigated in preclinical models and clinical trials to enhance tumor senescence and maximize efficacy against previously resistant NF1-driven tumors, such as MPNST.

Further clinical experience will also help refine and expand the use of MEK inhibition in NF1 and other RASopathies. Current studies are investigating alternative treatment schedules and treatment duration to determine if toxicities can be minimized for some patients. Also, long-term follow-up of clinical trials will help inform the understanding of potential late toxicities of MEK inhibition and whether there is an effect of age on toxicity, to better inform patients and families about risks of therapy. Finally, future clinical trials are needed to demonstrate how MEK inhibitors, and possibly other RAS-MAPK pathway inhibitors, can be safely and effectively used in other NF1 manifestations and related RASopathies.

MEK inhibitors provide the first FDA-approved therapy for NF1-driven PN and may be effective in the treatment of multiple other NF1-associated manifestations and other RASopathy manifestations. Although more study is required, the development of MEK inhibitors has already shed new light on the biology, treatment, and clinical care of common manifestations of NF1.

CLINICS CARE POINTS

- NF1 is the most common cancer predisposition syndrome; many tumors in individuals with NF1 affect young children and cause significant morbidity and mortality.

- MEK inhibitors are efficacious in the treatment of pediatric low-grade gliomas and plexiform neurofibromas. Selumetinib (an oral MEK inhibitor) is now FDA approved for use in children with inoperable plexiform neurofibromas.
- Although MEK inhibitors are well tolerated in children, ongoing surveillance for serious toxicities is required. Additional studies are ongoing to identify a modified schedule of administration to reduce the risk of toxicity.
- Combination therapy of MEK inhibitors with other treatment strategies is under preclinical and clinical investigation in the treatment of MPNST, because monotherapy with MEK inhibition is not effective for disease control.

DISCLOSURE

N. Ratner has awards from Revolution Medicine and Boehringer Ingelheim, unrelated to this article. P. de Blank has served on the pediatric oncology advisory board for Alexion Pharmaceuticals.

SUPPORT

N. Ratner is supported by NIH R01 awards NS12082, NS115438, NS028840, NIH R33 NS112407, and DOD W81XWH-19-1-0816.

REFERENCES

1. Kallionpaa RA, Uusitalo E, Leppavirta J, et al. Prevalence of neurofibromatosis type 1 in the Finnish population. Genet Med 2018;20(9):1082–6.
2. Kehrer-Sawatzki H, Cooper DN. Challenges in the diagnosis of neurofibromatosis type 1 (NF1) in children facilitated by means of revised diagnostic criteria including genetic testing for pathogenic NF1 gene variants. Hum Genet 2022; 141(2):177–91.
3. Legius E, Messiaen L, Wolkenstein P, et al. Revised diagnostic criteria for neurofibromatosis type 1 and Legius syndrome: an international consensus recommendation. Genet Med 2021;23(8):1506–13.
4. North KN, Riccardi V, Samango-Sprouse C, et al. Cognitive function and academic performance in neurofibromatosis. 1: consensus statement from the NF1 Cognitive Disorders Task Force. Neurology 1997;48(4):1121–7.
5. Lasater EA, Li F, Bessler WK, et al. Genetic and cellular evidence of vascular inflammation in neurofibromin-deficient mice and humans. J Clin Invest 2010; 120(3):859–70.
6. Sabbagh A, Pasmant E, Imbard A, et al. NF1 molecular characterization and neurofibromatosis type I genotype-phenotype correlation: the French experience. Hum Mutat 2013;34(11):1510–8.
7. Messiaen L, Yao S, Brems H, et al. Clinical and mutational spectrum of neurofibromatosis type 1-like syndrome. JAMA 2009;302(19):2111–8.
8. Riva M, Martorana D, Uliana V, et al. Recurrent NF1 gene variants and their genotype/phenotype correlations in patients with neurofibromatosis type I. Genes Chromosomes Cancer 2022;61(1):10–21.
9. Rice FL, Houk G, Wymer JP, et al. The evolution and multi-molecular properties of NF1 cutaneous neurofibromas originating from C-fiber sensory endings and terminal Schwann cells at normal sites of sensory terminations in the skin. PLoS One 2019;14(5):e0216527.

10. Serra E, Rosenbaum T, Nadal M, et al. Mitotic recombination effects homozygosity for NF1 germline mutations in neurofibromas. Nat Genet 2001;28(3):294–6.

11. Fisher MJ, Jones DTW, Li Y, et al. Integrated molecular and clinical analysis of low-grade gliomas in children with neurofibromatosis type 1 (NF1). Acta Neuropathol 2021;141(4):605–17.

12. Packer RJ, Iavarone A, Jones DTW, et al. Implications of new understandings of gliomas in children and adults with NF1: report of a consensus conference. Neuro Oncol 2020;22(6):773–84.

13. Gutmann DH, McLellan MD, Hussain I, et al. Somatic neurofibromatosis type 1 (NF1) inactivation characterizes NF1-associated pilocytic astrocytoma. Genome Res 2013;23(3):431–9.

14. Dombi E, Solomon J, Gillespie AJ, et al. NF1 plexiform neurofibroma growth rate by volumetric MRI: relationship to age and body weight. Neurology 2007;68(9): 643–7.

15. Kluwe L, Friedrich R, Mautner VF. Loss of NF1 allele in Schwann cells but not in fibroblasts derived from an NF1-associated neurofibroma. Genes Chromosomes Cancer 1999;24(3):283–5.

16. Korfhage J, Lombard DB. Malignant peripheral nerve sheath tumors: from epigenome to bedside. Mol Cancer Res 2019;17(7):1417–28.

17. Harder A. MEK inhibitors: novel targeted therapies of neurofibromatosis associated benign and malignant lesions. Biomark Res 2021;9(1):26.

18. Landry JP, Schertz KL, Chiang YJ, et al. Comparison of cancer prevalence in patients with neurofibromatosis type 1 at an academic cancer center vs in the general population from 1985 to 2020. JAMA Netw Open 2021;4(3):e210945.

19. Peltonen S, Kallionpaa RA, Rantanen M, et al. Pediatric malignancies in neurofibromatosis type 1: a population-based cohort study. Int J Cancer 2019;145(11): 2926–32.

20. Longo JF, Carroll SL. The RASopathies: biology, genetics and therapeutic options. Adv Cancer Res 2022;153:305–41.

21. Tidyman WE, Rauen KA. The RASopathies: developmental syndromes of Ras/MAPK pathway dysregulation. Curr Opin Genet Dev 2009;19(3):230–6.

22. Bos JL, Rehmann H, Wittinghofer A. GEFs and GAPs: critical elements in the control of small G proteins. Cell 2007;129(5):865–77.

23. Chang F, Steelman LS, Lee JT, et al. Signal transduction mediated by the Ras/Raf/MEK/ERK pathway from cytokine receptors to transcription factors: potential targeting for therapeutic intervention. Leukemia 2003;17(7):1263–93.

24. Chiariello M, Vaque JP, Crespo P, et al. Activation of Ras and Rho GTPases and MAP kinases by G-protein-coupled receptors. Methods Mol Biol 2010;661: 137–50.

25. Simanshu DK, Nissley DV, McCormick F. RAS proteins and their regulators in human disease. Cell 2017;170(1):17–33.

26. Arthur JS, Ley SC. Mitogen-activated protein kinases in innate immunity. Nat Rev Immunol 2013;13(9):679–92.

27. Brems H, Chmara M, Sahbatou M, et al. Germline loss-of-function mutations in SPRED1 cause a neurofibromatosis 1-like phenotype. Nat Genet 2007;39(9): 1120–6.

28. Yan W, Markegard E, Dharmaiah S, et al. Structural insights into the SPRED1-neurofibromin-KRAS complex and disruption of SPRED1-neurofibromin interaction by oncogenic EGFR. Cell Rep 2020;32(3):107909.

29. Lupton CJ, Bayly-Jones C, D'Andrea L, et al. The cryo-EM structure of the human neurofibromin dimer reveals the molecular basis for neurofibromatosis type 1. Nat Struct Mol Biol 2021;28(12):982–8.

30. Naschberger A, Baradaran R, Rupp B, et al. The structure of neurofibromin isoform 2 reveals different functional states. Nature 2021;599(7884):315–9.

31. Scheffzek K, Welti S. Neurofibromin: protein domains and functional characteristics. In: Upadhyaya M, Cooper DN, editors. Neurofibromatosis type 1: Molecular and cellular biology. Berlin, Heidelberg: Springer Berlin Heidelberg; 2012. p. 305–26.

32. Cichowski K, Shih TS, Schmitt E, et al. Mouse models of tumor development in neurofibromatosis type 1. Science 1999;286(5447):2172–6.

33. Jacks T, Shih TS, Schmitt EM, et al. Tumour predisposition in mice heterozygous for a targeted mutation in Nf1. Nat Genet 1994;7(3):353–61.

34. Zhu Y, Ghosh P, Charnay P, et al. Neurofibromas in NF1: Schwann cell origin and role of tumor environment. Science 2002;296(5569):920–2.

35. Wu J, Williams JP, Rizvi TA, et al. Plexiform and dermal neurofibromas and pigmentation are caused by Nf1 loss in desert hedgehog-expressing cells. Cancer Cell 2008;13(2):105–16.

36. Chen Z, Mo J, Brosseau JP, et al. Spatiotemporal loss of NF1 in Schwann cell lineage leads to different types of cutaneous neurofibroma susceptible to modification by the Hippo pathway. Cancer Discov 2019;9(1):114–29.

37. Radomska KJ, Coulpier F, Gresset A, et al. Cellular origin, tumor progression, and pathogenic mechanisms of cutaneous neurofibromas revealed by mice with Nf1 knockout in boundary cap cells. Cancer Discov 2019;9(1):130–47.

38. Prada CE, Jousma E, Rizvi TA, et al. Neurofibroma-associated macrophages play roles in tumor growth and response to pharmacological inhibition. Acta Neuropathol 2013;125(1):159–68.

39. Ribeiro S, Napoli I, White IJ, et al. Injury signals cooperate with Nf1 loss to relieve the tumor-suppressive environment of adult peripheral nerve. Cell Rep 2013;5(1):126–36.

40. Kershner LJ, Choi K, Wu J, et al. Multiple Nf1 Schwann cell populations reprogram the plexiform neurofibroma tumor microenvironment. JCI Insight 2022;7(18):e154513.

41. Widemann BC, Dombi E, Gillespie A, et al. Phase 2 randomized, flexible crossover, double-blinded, placebo-controlled trial of the farnesyltransferase inhibitor tipifarnib in children and young adults with neurofibromatosis type 1 and progressive plexiform neurofibromas. Neuro Oncol 2014;16(5):707–18.

42. Dombi E, Ardern-Holmes SL, Babovic-Vuksanovic D, et al. Recommendations for imaging tumor response in neurofibromatosis clinical trials. Neurology 2013;81(21 Suppl 1):S33–40.

43. Wu J, Dombi E, Jousma E, et al. Preclincial testing of sorafenib and RAD001 in the Nf(flox/flox); DhhCre mouse model of plexiform neurofibroma using magnetic resonance imaging. Pediatr Blood Cancer 2012;58(2):173–80.

44. Dombi E, Baldwin A, Marcus LJ, et al. Activity of selumetinib in neurofibromatosis type 1-related plexiform neurofibromas. N Engl J Med 2016;375(26):2550–60.

45. Jessen WJ, Miller SJ, Jousma E, et al. MEK inhibition exhibits efficacy in human and mouse neurofibromatosis tumors. J Clin Invest 2013;123(1):340–7.

46. Jousma E, Rizvi TA, Wu J, et al. Preclinical assessments of the MEK inhibitor PD-0325901 in a mouse model of neurofibromatosis type 1. Pediatr Blood Cancer 2015;62(10):1709–16.

47. Robertson KA, Nalepa G, Yang FC, et al. Imatinib mesylate for plexiform neuro-fibromas in patients with neurofibromatosis type 1: a phase 2 trial. Lancet Oncol 2012;13(12):1218–24.

48. Casey D, Demko S, Sinha A, et al. FDA approval summary: selumetinib for plex-iform neurofibroma. Clin Cancer Res 2021;27(15):4142–6.

49. Gross AM, Wolters PL, Dombi E, et al. Selumetinib in children with inoperable plexiform neurofibromas. N Engl J Med 2020;382(15):1430–42.

50. Weiss BD, Wolters PL, Plotkin SR, et al. NF106: a Neurofibromatosis Clinical Trials Consortium phase II trial of the MEK inhibitor mirdametinib (PD-0325901) in ad-olescents and adults with NF1-related plexiform neurofibromas. J Clin Oncol 2021;39(7):797–806.

51. Fisher MJ, Shih CS, Rhodes SD, et al. Cabozantinib for neurofibromatosis type 1-related plexiform neurofibromas: a phase 2 trial. Nat Med 2021;27(1):165–73.

52. Fangusaro J, Onar-Thomas A, Young Poussaint T, et al. Selumetinib in paediatric patients with BRAF-aberrant or neurofibromatosis type 1-associated recurrent, refractory, or progressive low-grade glioma: a multicentre, phase 2 trial. Lancet Oncol 2019;20(7):1011–22.

53. Stieglitz E, Taylor-Weiner AN, Chang TY, et al. The genomic landscape of juvenile myelomonocytic leukemia. Nat Genet 2015;47(11):1326–33.

54. Gupta AK, Meena JP, Chopra A, et al. Juvenile myelomonocytic leukemia: a comprehensive review and recent advances in management. Am J Blood Res 2021;11(1):1–21.

55. Lyubynska N, Gorman MF, Lauchle JO, et al. A MEK inhibitor abrogates myelo-proliferative disease in Kras mutant mice. Sci Transl Med 2011;3(76):76ra27.

56. Kolberg M, Holand M, Agesen TH, et al. Survival meta-analyses for >1800 malig-nant peripheral nerve sheath tumor patients with and without neurofibromatosis type 1. Neuro Oncol 2013;15(2):135–47.

57. Ma Y, Gross AM, Dombi E, et al. A molecular basis for neurofibroma-associated skeletal manifestations in NF1. Genet Med 2020;22(11):1786–93.

58. Rios JJ, Richards BS, Stevenson DA, et al. Are some randomized clinical trials impossible? J Pediatr Orthop 2021;41(1):e90–3.

59. Hyman SL, Shores A, North KN. The nature and frequency of cognitive deficits in children with neurofibromatosis type 1. Neurology 2005;65(7):1037–44.

60. Schwetye KE, Gutmann DH. Cognitive and behavioral problems in children with neurofibromatosis type 1: challenges and future directions. Expert Rev Neurother 2014;14(10):1139–52.

61. Walsh KS, Wolters PL, Widemann BC, et al. Impact of MEK inhibitor therapy on neurocognitive functioning in NF1. Neurol Genet 2021;7(5):e616.

62. Lalancette E, Cantin E, Routhier M-E, et al. Impact of trametinib on the neuropsy-chological profile of NF1 patients. Annual Meeting of the Children's Tumor Foun-dation; 2022.

63. de Blank PMK, Gross AM, Akshintala S, et al. MEK inhibitors for neurofibroma-tosis type 1 manifestations: clinical evidence and consensus. Neuro Oncol 2022;24(11):1845–56.

64. Bobyn JD, Deo N, Little DG, et al. Modulation of spine fusion with BMP-2, MEK inhibitor (PD0325901), and zoledronic acid in a murine model of NF1 double inac-tivation. J Orthop Sci 2021;26(4):684–9.

65. Klesse LJ, Jordan JT, Radtke HB, et al. The use of MEK inhibitors in neurofibro-matosis type 1-associated tumors and management of toxicities. Oncol 2020; 25(7):e1109–16.

66. Aoki Y, Niihori T, Narumi Y, et al. The RAS/MAPK syndromes: novel roles of the RAS pathway in human genetic disorders. Hum Mutat 2008;29(8):992–1006.
67. Niemeyer CM. RAS diseases in children. Haematologica 2014;99(11):1653–62.
68. Dori Y, Smith C, Pinto E, et al. Severe lymphatic disorder resolved with MEK inhibition in a patient with Noonan syndrome and SOS1 mutation. Pediatrics 2020; 146(6):e20200167.
69. Nakano TA, Rankin AW, Annam A, et al. Trametinib for refractory chylous effusions and systemic complications in children with Noonan syndrome. J Pediatr 2022; 248:81–88 e81.
70. Andelfinger G, Marquis C, Raboisson MJ, et al. Hypertrophic cardiomyopathy in Noonan syndrome treated by MEK-inhibition. J Am Coll Cardiol 2019;73(17): 2237–9.
71. Leegaard A, Gregersen PA, Nielsen TO, et al. Successful MEK-inhibition of severe hypertrophic cardiomyopathy in RIT1-related Noonan syndrome. Eur J Med Genet 2022;65(11):104630.

Shedding New Light

Novel Therapies for Achondroplasia and Growth Disorders

Nadia Merchant, MD[a,b],*, Andrew Dauber, MD, MMSc[a,b]

KEYWORDS

- Achondroplasia • *FGFR3* • Skeletal dysplasia • Treatment • Short stature
- Growth disorders precision medicine

KEY POINTS

- Achondroplasia is the most common form of skeletal dysplasia which results in dispropor-tionate severe short stature due to heterozygous gain-of-function variants of the fibroblast growth factor receptor 3 (*FGFR3*) gene that inhibits endochondral ossification.
- Management of achondroplasia has been largely symptomatic for potential medical com-plications and psychosocial implications.
- There are multiple novel therapeutic approaches for achondroplasia on the horizon.
- Vosoritide, a C-type natriuretic peptide analog, is currently approved in the US (age >5 years), in Europe, Brazil, and Australia (age >2 years), and in Japan (all ages) for the treatment of achondroplasia in children whose growth plates are not closed.
- Long-term data on the effects of pharmacotherapies on medical comorbidities in achon-droplasia are pending at this time.

INTRODUCTION

Achondroplasia is the most common form of skeletal dysplasia which results in dispro-portionate severe short stature.[1] There is an estimated incidence of approximately 1 in 10,000-30,000 live births.[1,2] There are more than 250,000 affected persons world-wide.[3] Achondroplasia is an autosomal dominant genetic disorder caused by hetero-zygous gain-of-function variants of the fibroblast growth factor receptor 3 (*FGFR3*) gene that inhibits endochondral ossification. Greater than 98% of patients with achon-droplasia have a heterozygous pathogenic variant in *FGFR3* with the same nucleotide change regardless of ethnicity. The pathogenic variant c.1138G>A (p.Gly380Arg) in

[a] Division of Endocrinology, Children's National Hospital, Washington, DC 20010, USA;
[b] Department of Pediatrics, George Washington University School of Medicine and Health Sciences, Washington, DC 20037, USA
* Corresponding author. Division of Endocrinology, Children's National Hospital, Washington, DC 20010.
E-mail address: nmerchant@childrensnational.org

Pediatr Clin N Am 70 (2023) 951–961
https://doi.org/10.1016/j.pcl.2023.05.008
0031-3955/23/© 2023 Elsevier Inc. All rights reserved.

pediatric.theclinics.com

approximately 98% and c.1138G>C (p.Gly380Arg) in approximately 1% of individuals are heterozygous achondroplasia. There is no recognized predisposition based on ethnicity or sex.[1] Over 80% of cases arise from *de novo* variants. Advanced paternal age is a known risk factor.[4] Since the majority are *de novo* variants, this means that 80% of patients with achondroplasia are born to average-stature parents.

Achondroplasia usually is diagnosed clinically based on specific clinical characteristics and features on radiographs. Clinical features include relative or absolute macrocephaly, midface hypoplasia with a short distance between eyebrows to mouth, flat nasal bridge, short nose and flat face, trident configuration of the hands, and disproportionate short stature with rhizomelia (proximal long bones) and near-normal length of the trunk with normal cognition. On a skeletal survey, a square-shaped pelvis with small sacrosciatic notch, short pedicles of the vertebrae with interpedicular narrowing from lower thoracic to the lumbar region, rhizomelia, proximal femoral radiolucency, and chevron shape of the distal femoral epiphysis can be appreciated. Molecular confirmation is not required for every child with achondroplasia but should be considered if there is an atypical presentation.[1] The average adult height in achondroplasia is 120-135 cm (4-4.5 feet), and it is recommended to use achondroplasia specific growth curves.[5] The growth velocity is about 4 cm/year in achondroplasia with length/height around −4 to −5 standard deviations (SD) in childhood and about −6 to −7 SD as adults due to lack of a significant growth spurt during puberty.[5]

There are currently 461 skeletal disorders classified into 42 groups with over 350 skeletal dysplasias known to cause short stature.[6] However, only a handful of conditions exist that may be confused with achondroplasia. An understanding of the growth plate is important in order to have a deeper understanding of the pathophysiology of skeletal dysplasias as well as potential treatment options.

PHYSIOLOGY AT THE GROWTH PLATE

The growth plate is a thin layer of cartilage found at the ends of long bones and vertebrae where longitudinal growth takes place.[7] Growth is regulated at the growth plate by a dynamic process called endochondral ossification that is controlled by multiple factors including hormones (eg, growth hormone, insulin-like growth factor-1, estrogen, androgens, thyroid, glucocorticoids) and interaction of receptors and signaling pathways (eg, FGFR3, CNP, MAPK).[8]

Endochondral ossification is the process in which cartilage is first formed by chondrocytes and then remodeled into bone tissue. The postnatal growth plate contains chondrocytes at different stages of differentiation that are separated into five layers. The chondrocytes pass through a stepwise process from resting to proliferative to prehypertrophic to hypertrophic to the terminal phase. The resting zone chondrocytes act as stem-like cells to replenish the proliferative chondrocytes and replicate at a slow rate compared to the proliferative zone.

With the advancement in genetics over the last few decades, there is now a greater understanding of paracrine factors secreted in the growth plate by chondrocytes. Variants in genes involved in paracrine signaling significantly impair growth in animal models and humans.[8] The gene *FGFR3* was found to be the cause of achondroplasia in 1994. It is located on chromosome 4p16.3. FGFR3 is one of the four closely related receptors for fibroblast growth factors that are present on cell membranes, most prominent on chondrocytes which make cartilage.[4] At the growth plate, FGFR3 signaling negatively regulates growth by decreasing proliferation in the proliferative zone, decreasing the production of extracellular matrix, accelerating the onset of hypertrophic differentiation, and decreasing the size of hypertrophic chondrocytes. FGFR3 is a tyrosine-kinase receptor that generally inhibits endochondral ossification downstream by activating STAT1 (signal transducer and activator of transcription 1) as well as the MAPK (mitogen-activated protein kinase) pathway through a signaling cascade involving RAS-RAF-MEK-ERK. The MAPK signaling negatively regulates chondrocyte proliferation and differentiation.[9,10] Another important growth factor, c-type natriuretic peptide (CNP) signals through its receptor, natriuretic peptide receptor 2 (NPR2), which leads to the inhibition of the MAPK pathway thereby promoting growth.[8]

Activating mutations in *FGFR3* impair linear growth in patients with achondroplasia, hypochondroplasia, and thanatophoric dysplasia.[7] Parathyroid hormone-related protein (PTHrP) maintains the width of the growth plate, hence variants in PTHrP can cause shortening of the proliferative zone, premature closure of the growth plate, and short stature.[7] Genetic defects that lead to overexpression of CNP or activating variants in *NPR2* lead to tall stature while variants inactivating *NPR2* lead to short stature.[8] Chondrocytes secrete aggrecan, which is a major proteoglycan component of the cartilage extracellular matrix. Aggrecan helps provide the resilience property of cartilage and plays a role in regulating chondrogenesis at the growth plate. Variants in the gene *ACAN*, encoding aggrecan, affect linear growth often resulting in advanced bone age and early cessation of growth.[7,8] Numerous other genetic defects in the growth plate can lead to skeletal dysplasias and growth disorders.[8]

FIBROBLAST GROWTH FACTOR RECEPTOR 3-RELATED GROWTH DISORDERS

Variants in the gene that encodes fibroblast growth factor receptor 3 (*FGFR3*) are associated with hypochondroplasia, achondroplasia, achondroplasia double dominant, and thanatophoric dysplasia.[11]

Hypochondroplasia

Patients with hypochondroplasia may appear normal at birth. They are characterized by macrocephaly, stocky build, mild joint laxity, disproportionately short arms and legs, and broad short hands and feet. The skeletal and radiological features are similar to achondroplasia but milder, with fewer medical complications such as obstructive sleep apnea and spinal stenosis. However, intellectual disability and epilepsy may be more prevalent.[12]

Thanatophoric Dysplasia

This condition is typically lethal in the perinatal period due to respiratory insufficiency shortly following birth. There are two clinically distinct forms, type I (80%) and type II (20%). Type I is characterized by micromelia with bowed femurs. Type II is characterized by micromelia with straight femurs and uniform presence of moderate-to-severe cloverleaf skull deformity. Both types have infantile hypotonia, macrocephaly, frontal bossing, flat facies with ocular proptosis, brachydactyly, and micromelia. TD is usually incidentally discovered or suspected during a routine prenatal ultrasound. Specific findings during the second and third-trimester ultrasounds include a cloverleaf skull, macrocephaly, ventriculomegaly, increased nuchal translucency, a narrow chest cavity with short ribs, and bowed femurs (TD type I). TD is also only caused by variants in *FGFR3*, and the pathogenic variant p.Lys650Glu has been identified in all diagnosed individuals with TD type II.[13,14]

Severe Achondroplasia with Developmental Delay and Acanthosis Nigricans

This is also due to variants in *FGFR3*. It is characterized by affected individuals developing extensive areas of acanthosis nigricans starting in early childhood, and they suffer from severe neurological impairments. On exam and imaging, they have femoral bowing, apex posterior tibial and fibular bowing, and curved "ram's horn" deformities of the clavicles.[15]

MANAGEMENT

Management of achondroplasia has been largely symptomatic. Potential medical complications include foramen magnum stenosis, hydrocephalus, upper airway obstruction, middle ear dysfunction, restrictive pulmonary disease, lower extremity long bone bowing, thoracolumbar kyphosis, and lumbosacral stenosis. There are age-specific recommendations, since there are well-known significant complications that may need early intervention with timely referrals to neurosurgery, otolaryngology, and orthopedics. Most individuals with achondroplasia have a normal life expectancy, however, mortality is increased in infants and young children due to hydrocephalus, sleep apnea, and sudden death related to foramen magnum stenosis.[16] As soon as an infant is diagnosed, neuroimaging is recommended to assess the craniocervical junction for narrowing, ventricle size, and amount of extra-axial cerebrospinal fluid (CSF). It is also important to obtain a regular detailed history and neurological exam for concerns related to sleep apnea, feeding difficulties, abnormal movements, cyanosis with feeding or sleeping, and to assess muscle tone. Achondroplasia-specific developmental charts should be used.[1] A sleep study should be done to assess for central or obstructive sleep apnea. There are also increased rates of middle ear problems and conductive hearing loss due to fluid buildup requiring tympanostomy tubes, hence it is recommended to perform an annual hearing evaluation. The spinal cord is normal in size with a small spinal canal, hence there is a risk for lumbosacral spinal stenosis. Complications of spinal stenosis include numbness, weakness, and altered deep tendon reflexes. Early intervention may lead to better outcomes. There are potential psychosocial implications for both the parents and child related to short stature. A multidisciplinary approach is needed to manage patients with achondroplasia. A recent international consensus statement and an American Academy of Pediatrics health supervision guidelines provide recommended anticipatory guidance, screening protocols, and management advice.[1,17]

Surgical interventions aim to improve specific complications: decompression surgeries for foramen magnum narrowing or spinal stenosis, tonsillectomy or adenoidectomy for obstructive sleep apnea, and tympanostomy tube insertion for recurrent otitis media. Surgical limb lengthening has been investigated since the 1930s for height and proportionality.[18] However, in practice, the use of limb lengthening varies by geography and can be associated with high treatment burden and severe complications.[1] Procedures are only performed on long bones, such as femur or tibia and therefore do not help with complications related to other bone types.[18]

Rare disease drugs are currently being studied for achondroplasia. The current drugs under investigation or recently approved to target the growth plate to stimulate chondrocyte differentiation and hypertrophy, including analogues of C-type natriuretic peptide (CNP), FGFR3-selective tyrosine kinase inhibitors, anti-FGFR3 antibodies, aptamers targeting FGF2, and soluble forms of FGFR3 are possible treatments for achondroplasia and other causes of short stature (**Fig. 1**).

PHARMACOTHERAPY
Growth Hormone

Growth hormone has been trialed as an intervention to improve height in children with achondroplasia. Currently, growth hormone is only approved in Japan for this

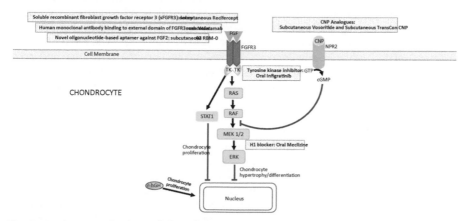

Fig. 1. At the growth plate of chondrocyte, FGF (fibroblast growth factor) acts on FGFR3 (fibroblast growth factor receptor 3) which activates RAS-MAPK pathway resulting in the inhibition of chondrocyte proliferation and differentiation. CNP (C-type natriuretic peptide) binds to its receptor, natriuretic peptide receptor 2 (gene NPR2) causing the transformation of GTP into cGMP leading to the inhibition of MAPK (mitogen-activated protein kinase) leading to chondrocyte hypertrophy and differentiation. rhGH leads to chondrocyte proliferation. There are drugs currently approved, under investigation or potential therapeutic agents at the level of the growth plate. This includes CNP analogues (Vosoritide and Trans-Con CNP), H1 blocker (meclizine), soluble recombinant human fibroblast growth factor receptor that binds to FGF (Recifercept), human monoclonal antibody binding to external domain of FGFR3 (Vofatamab), novel oligonucleotide-based aptamer against FGF2 (RBM-007) and tyrosine kinase inhibitor selectivity for the FGFR receptor family (Infigratinib).

indication. It was approved based on a height gain of 1-1.5 SD at a supraphysiologic growth hormone dose of 0.05 mg/kg/day.[19] After 6 years of treatment, a gain of adult height in males was 3.5-8 cm and in females was 2.8-4.2 cm with most of the gain in the first few years. The long-term efficacy and use of growth hormone in achondroplasia have been debated, and it is not widely used around the world.[20]

C-type Natriuretic Peptide

Paracrine factor C-type natriuretic peptide (CNP) signals through its receptor encoded by the natriuretic peptide receptor 2 (*NPR2*) gene leading to the inhibition of the ERK/MAPK pathway which is downstream of FGFR3. Native CNP has a short half-life of 2-3 minutes as it is degraded by neutral-endopeptidase proteolysis (NEP). There are currently two forms of CNP analogs: Vosoritide and TansCon CNP.

Vosoritide

Vosoritide (BMN 111) is a small molecule peptide (CNP analog) that mimics CNP activity with an extended half-life as a result of neutral-endopeptidase proteolysis resistance that allows for once-daily subcutaneous administration. In juvenile, skeletally normal mice and monkeys, administration of once-daily subcutaneous recombinant CNP analog, promoted long-bone growth that was hemodynamically tolerable.[21] Mouse models with a skeletal phenotype of achondroplasia due to increased activation of *FGFR3* had improved long-bone and craniofacial growth after receiving vosoritide.[21,22] This led to a multinational, Phase 2, open-label, safety and dose finding trial with a total of 35 children with achondroplasia between the ages of 5 and 14 years who received vosoritide once-daily subcutaneously at 4 different dosages. The study demonstrated that the side-effect profile is generally mild and treatment with daily vosoritide at the two highest doses (15 µg/kg/daily and 30 µg/kg/daily) led to sustained increases in the annualized height velocity for up to 42 months.[23] The most common treatment-related adverse events were transient injection-site reactions and mild changes in blood pressure that were self-limited. A secondary outcome looked at markers of bone growth and CNP activity. There was a dose-dependent increase in urinary cGMP (biomarker of drug activity) and an increase in a biomarker of endochondral ossification, serum collage X marker (CXM), with maximum response in those receiving the 15- and 30-mcg/kg doses.[23] This was followed by a Phase 3, randomized, double-blind, placebo-controlled trial in children with achondroplasia with age range 5 to <18 years from seven countries with 60 subjects assigned to receive 15 µg/kg/daily of vosoritide and 61 subjects to receive a placebo. The primary outcome was the adjusted mean difference in annualized height velocity after 52 weeks between patients in the vosoritide group and placebo group. Subjects in the vosoritide group had an annualized height velocity that was 1.57 cm/year higher compared to placebo with no serious adverse events.[24,25] Secondary outcomes included changes in the upper-to-lower segment ratio by calculating the ratio between sitting height and standing height minus sitting height, safety and tolerability of vosoritide, and changes in CXM. In the first year of this study, there was no difference in the incidence of side effects between treated and control groups, and no-drug related serious adverse events including cardiovascular issues. In the phase 3 extension study, analysis on the upper-to-lower body segment ratio showed a statistically significant greater decrease in body ratio in vosoritide treated versus the untreated group and change in height Z-score (95% CI) was +0.44 (0.25, 0.63) at week 104.[24] Vosoritide was approved in children with achondroplasia in the European Union and Brazil for age greater than two years and United States of America for age greater than five years in 2021 till growth plates fuse; approved in Australia for ages greater than two and Japan after birth in 2022 till growth plates fuse.

TransCon C-type natriuretic peptide

TransCon CNP is a C-type natriuretic peptide conjugated via a cleavable linker to a polyethylene glycol carrier molecule that allows for sustained systemic CNP levels with weekly subcutaneous administration. TransCon CNP has almost complete resistance to NEP. The half-life in monkeys and humans is approximately 90 hours. In mice and cynomolgus monkeys, sustained exposure to CNP provided by TransCon CNP was more efficacious in stimulating bone growth than intermittent CNP exposure.[26] The body length was increased by 5% and tail length by 3% for those treated with TransCon CNP and body length increased by 3% and tail length 3% compared with the observed growth in control monkeys.[26] In a mouse model of achondroplasia, there was growth of tibia, femur, and spine with the injection of TransCon CNP that was comparable to results in published data of mice receiving vosoritide.[26] A Phase 1 trial has been completed supporting that TransCon CNP is well tolerated with a pharmacokinetic profile appropriate for a once-weekly dosing regimen. Plasma and urine levels of cGMP were significantly increased in subjects administered TransCon CNP at 75-150 µg CNP/kg, indicating CNP activity at its receptor for at least 1-week post-dose. It was well-tolerated with no serious treatment-emergent adverse events or discontinuations.[9] Currently, there is a phase 2, multicenter, double-blind, randomized, placebo control, dose-escalation trial to determine the safety, efficacy, and pharmacokinetics of once weekly subcutaneous doses of TransCon CNP for prepubertal children between 2 and 10 years of age which is ongoing.[27]

Infigratinib: FGFR1-3 Inhibitor

Infigratinib is an orally bioavailable tyrosine kinase inhibitor (TKI) that selectively targets FGFR1-3.[28] On May 28, 2021, the Food and Drug Administration granted accelerated approval to infigratinib for adults with previously treated, unresectable locally advanced or metastatic cholangiocarcinoma with a fibroblast growth factor receptor 2 (FGFR2) fusion or other rearrangement.[29] Infigratinib counteracts FGFR3 hyperactivity by reducing FGFR3 phosphorylation and downstream signaling. It was shown to correct abnormal femoral growth plate in organ cultures in the $Fgfr3^{Y367C/+}$ mouse model of achondroplasia. Low dose Infigratinib injected subcutaneously was able to penetrate the growth plate and modify its organization in the $Fgfr3^{Y367C/+}$ mice. It inhibited *FGFR3* downstream signaling pathways including *MAPK, SOX9, STAT1* in the growth plates of $Fgfr3^{Y367C/+}$ mice and in cultured chondrocyte models of ACH.[30] Infigratinib treatment led to a greater growth effect than seen with vosoritide treatment in $Fgfr3^{Y367C/+}$ mice.[30] A prospective, multicenter, phase II, open-label study of infigratinib in children with achondroplasia is ongoing. The initial study included dose escalation of four doses to characterize the pharmacokinetic (PK) profile of infigratinib and explore safety and preliminary efficacy.[28] A press release announced that the cohort receiving the highest dose (0.128 mg/kg once daily) had a mean increase of annualized growth velocity of 1.52 cm/year in children 5 years of age and older and it was well-tolerated with no serious adverse events and no discontinuations due to adverse events. Based on this, another cohort was added to receive higher dosing of infigratinib (0.25 mg/kg daily).[31]

Recifercept: FGFR3 Decoy

Recifercept is a recombinant protein, a soluble form of the human FGFR3 (sFGFR3) that acts as a decoy receptor and prevents FGF from binding to FGFR3. The extracellular domain of FGFR3 requires binding by FGFs to induce signaling. Recifercept is thought to act as a ligand to trap FGFs, hence preventing the activation of FGFR3 thereby preventing downstream signaling. This results in blocking the negative growth signal which allows increased cell proliferation. Recifercept binds to FGF isoforms *in vitro*, and in cellular model systems, it reduces FGFR3 signaling. In a transgenic $Fgfr3^{Y367C/+}$ mouse model of achondroplasia, sFGFR3 improved long bone growth after administering twice per week subcutaneous injections for three weeks during the growth period. Mice treated with recifercept showed similar body proportions to wild-type without any evidence of complications from treatment.[32] After completing phase 2 multiple dose, randomized study for 12 months to assess the safety, tolerability, pharmacokinetics, and efficacy of subcutaneous Recifercept in children with achondroplasia, decision was made to terminate any further clinical trials.[33]

Meclizine: H1 Blocker

Through a drug repositioning strategy, oral meclizine was identified to suppress FGFR3 signaling in three different chondrocyte cell lines and embryonic bone organ culture.[10] Meclizine dihydrochloride is an anti-histamine drug that is FDA approved for motion sickness. Analyses of intracellular FGFR3 signaling showed that meclizine downregulates the FGFR3 signaling by possibly attenuating extracellular-signal-regulated kinase (ERK) phosphorylation. Meclizine was as efficient as CNP in attenuating the abnormal FGFR3 signaling in chondrocyte cell lines.[10] Bone lengths and vertebrae were significantly longer in meclizine-treated $Fgfr3^{ach}$ mice compared to untreated $Fgfr3^{ach}$ mice.[34] The short stature phenotype in the $Fgfr3^{ach}$ mice was significantly decreased by twice-daily oral administration of 2 mg/kg/day of meclizine. This dose, based on pharmacokinetic analyses, demonstrated that peak drug concentration (Cmax) and area under the concentration-time curve (AUC) of 2 mg/kg of meclizine in mice was lower than that of 25 mg/body to humans that is used for anti-motion-sickness.[35] A phase Ia study on twelve children with achondroplasia from age 5 to 11 years of age has been conducted to evaluate the pharmacokinetics and safety of meclizine. The first six subjects received once a day meclizine while fasting and the other six children received it twice a day with no serious adverse events for 14 days. The plasma concentration reached a steady state around 10 days after the first dose with once a day and twice a day dosing.[36] Additional studies are ongoing to further investigate meclizine as a therapeutic option in achondroplasia.

RBM-007: Aptamer Against FGFR2

RBM-007 is a FGF2–targeting RNA aptamer that prevents FGF2 from activating FGFR3. In rat chondrocytes and mouse tibia organ cultures, chondrocyte proliferation and differentiation were improved with RBM-007. Subcutaneous administration of the aptamer also restored bone growth in a mouse model of achondroplasia.[37] A phase I study has been completed to evaluate the safety, tolerability, and pharmacokinetics of RBM-007. In Japan, there is currently a phase 2 study being conducted.[38]

Vofatamab: Human Monoclonal Antibody Binding to the External Domain of FGF3

Vofatamab is a human IgG1 monoclonal antibody that specifically binds to FGFR3. *FGFR3* gain of function variants is known to be found in a variety of cancers, including multiple myeloma and urothelial cell carcinoma. At this time, there are no preclinical studies for Vofatamab published for achondroplasia.[39]

DISCUSSION

With the advancement in genetics, there is now a greater understanding of the underlying pathophysiology of skeletal dysplasias and growth disorders. An understanding of the growth plate has led to the discovery of potential treatment options for achondroplasia that is now beyond symptomatic management. Rare disease drugs are currently being studied for achondroplasia with the hope to improve growth and reduce complications. Vosoritide is currently approved in the US (age >5 years), in Europe, Brazil, and Australia (age >2 years), and in Japan (all ages) for the treatment of achondroplasia in children whose growth plates are not closed. Long-term data on the effects of these therapies on medical comorbidities are pending at this time. Multiple other novel therapeutic approaches show promise and the possibility of combined therapies may reduce medical complications if the medications can be started at an early age. While these drugs are being developed for achondroplasia, they may have therapeutic benefits in other skeletal dysplasias and growth disorders. We are currently conducting a clinical trial of vosoritide in selected genetic disorders including hypochondroplasia, Rasopathies, SHOX deficiency, *ACAN* gene variants, *NPPC,* and *NPR2* gene variants.[40]

SUMMARY

Achondroplasia is the most common form of skeletal dysplasia which results in disproportionate severe short stature. Management of achondroplasia has been largely symptomatic for medical complications and psychosocial implications. There are multiple novel pharmacotherapies on the horizon for achondroplasia.

CLINICS CARE POINTS

- Achondroplasia is the most common form of skeletal dysplasia which results in disproportionate severe short stature due to heterozygous gain-of-function variants of the fibroblast growth factor receptor 3 (*FGFR3*) gene that inhibits endochondral ossification.

- Management of achondroplasia has been largely symptomatic for potential medical complications including foramen magnum stenosis, lower extremity long bone bowing, middle ear dysfunction, thoracolumbar kyphosis, and spinal stenosis.

- There are multiple novel therapeutic approaches for achondroplasia on the horizon.

- Vosoritide is currently approved in the US (age >5 years), in Europe, Brazil, and Australia (age >2 years), and in Japan (all ages) for the treatment of achondroplasia in children whose growth plates are not closed. Long-term data on the effects of these therapies on medical comorbidities are pending at this time.

DISCLOSURE

A. Dauber has current research support from BioMarin. He has served as a consultant for BioMarin, Pfizer, Ascendis, QED Therapeutics, and Novo Nordisk. N. Merchant has served as a consultant for BioMarin and Pfizer.

REFERENCES

1. Hoover-Fong J, Scott CI, Jones MC, Committee On G. Health supervision for people with achondroplasia. Pediatrics 2020;145(6). https://doi.org/10.1542/peds. 2020-1010.
2. Foreman PK, van Kessel F, van Hoorn R, et al. Birth prevalence of achondroplasia: a systematic literature review and meta-analysis. Am J Med Genet 2020;182(10):2297–316.
3. Ireland PJ, Pacey V, Zankl A, et al. Optimal management of complications associated with achondroplasia. Appl Clin Genet 2014;7:117–25.
4. Horton WA, Hall JG, Hecht JT. Achondroplasia. Lancet (London, England) 2007; 370(9582):162–72.
5. Hoover-Fong JE, Schulze KJ, Alade AY, et al. Growth in achondroplasia including stature, weight, weight-for-height and head circumference from CLARITY: achondroplasia natural history study-a multi-center retrospective cohort study of achondroplasia in the US. Orphanet J Rare Dis 2021;16(1):522.
6. Mortier GR, Cohn DH, Cormier-Daire V, et al. Nosology and classification of genetic skeletal disorders: 2019 revision. Am J Med Genet 2019;179(12):2393–419.
7. Allen DB, Merchant N, Miller BS, et al. Evolution and future of growth plate therapeutics. Horm Res Paediatr 2021;94(9–10):319–32.
8. Baron J, Savendahl L, De Luca F, et al. Short and tall stature: a new paradigm emerges. Nat Rev Endocrinol 2015;11(12):735–46.
9. Breinholt VM, Mygind PH, Christoffersen ED, et al. Phase 1 safety, tolerability, pharmacokinetics and pharmacodynamics results of a long-acting C-type natriuretic peptide prodrug, TransCon CNP. Br J Clin Pharmacol 2022. https://doi. org/10.1111/bcp.15369.
10. Matsushita M, Kitoh H, Ohkawara B, et al. Meclozine facilitates proliferation and differentiation of chondrocytes by attenuating abnormally activated FGFR3 signaling in achondroplasia. PLoS One 2013;8(12):e81569.

11. Almeida MR, Campos-Xavier AB, Medeira A, et al. Clinical and molecular diagnosis of the skeletal dysplasias associated with mutations in the gene encoding Fibroblast Growth Factor Receptor 3 (FGFR3) in Portugal. Clin Genet 2009;75(2):150–6.

12. Bober MB, Bellus GA, Nikkel SM, et al. Hypochondroplasia. 1999 Jul 15 [Updated 2020 May 7]. In: Adam MP, Mirzaa GM, Pagon RA, et al. editors. GeneReviews® [Internet]. Seattle (WA): University of Washington, Seattle; 1993-2023. Available at: https://www.ncbi.nlm.nih.gov/books/NBK1477/.

13. French T, Savarirayan R. Thanatophoric Dysplasia. 2004 May 21 [Updated 2023 May 18]. In: Adam MP, Mirzaa GM, Pagon RA, et al. editors. GeneReviews® [Internet]. Seattle (WA): University of Washington, Seattle; 1993-2023. Available at: https://www.ncbi.nlm.nih.gov/books/NBK1366/.

14. Jimah BB, Mensah TA, Ulzen-Appiah K, et al. Prenatal diagnosis of skeletal dysplasia and review of the literature. Case Rep Obstet Gynecol 2021;2021:9940063.

15. Tavormina PL, Bellus GA, Webster MK, et al. A novel skeletal dysplasia with developmental delay and acanthosis nigricans is caused by a Lys650Met mutation in the fibroblast growth factor receptor 3 gene. Am J Hum Genet 1999;64(3):722–31.

16. Wynn J, King TM, Gambello MJ, et al. Mortality in achondroplasia study: a 42-year follow-up. Am J Med Genet 2007;143A(21):2502–11.

17. Savarirayan R, Ireland P, Irving M, et al. International Consensus Statement on the diagnosis, multidisciplinary management and lifelong care of individuals with achondroplasia. Nat Rev Endocrinol 2022;18(3):173–89.

18. Hosny GA. Limb lengthening history, evolution, complications and current concepts. J Orthop Trauma 2020;21(1):3.

19. Yorifuji T, Higuchi S, Kawakita R. Growth hormone treatment for achondroplasia. Pediatr Endocrinol Rev 2018;16(Suppl 1):123–8.

20. Miccoli M, Bertelloni S, Massart F. Height outcome of recombinant human growth hormone treatment in achondroplasia children: a meta-analysis. Horm Res Paediatr 2016;86(1):27–34.

21. Wendt DJ, Dvorak-Ewell M, Bullens S, et al. Neutral endopeptidase-resistant C-type natriuretic peptide variant represents a new therapeutic approach for treatment of fibroblast growth factor receptor 3-related dwarfism. J Pharmacol Exp Ther 2015;353(1):132–49.

22. Lorget F, Kaci N, Peng J, et al. Evaluation of the therapeutic potential of a CNP analog in a Fgfr3 mouse model recapitulating achondroplasia. Am J Hum Genet 2012;91(6):1108–14.

23. Savarirayan R, Irving M, Bacino CA, et al. C-type natriuretic peptide analogue therapy in children with achondroplasia. N Engl J Med 2019;381(1):25–35.

24. Savarirayan R, Tofts L, Irving M, et al. Safe and persistent growth-promoting effects of vosoritide in children with achondroplasia: 2-year results from an open-label, phase 3 extension study. Genet Med 2021;23(12):2443–7.

25. Savarirayan R, Tofts L, Irving M, et al. Once-daily, subcutaneous vosoritide therapy in children with achondroplasia: a randomised, double-blind, phase 3, placebo-controlled, multicentre trial. Lancet (London, England) 2020;396(10252):684–92.

26. Breinholt VM, Rasmussen CE, Mygind PH, et al. TransCon CNP, a sustained-release C-type natriuretic peptide prodrug, a potentially safe and efficacious new therapeutic modality for the treatment of comorbidities associated with fibroblast growth factor receptor 3-related skeletal dysplasias. J Pharmacol Exp Ther 2019;370(3):459–71.

27. Available at: https://clinicaltrials.gov/ct2/show/NCT05246033?cond=achondroplasia&draw=2&rank=2. Accessed June 25, 2023.

28. Savarirayan R, De Bergua JM, Arundel P, et al. Infigratinib in children with achondroplasia: the PROPEL and PROPEL 2 studies. Ther Adv Musculoskelet Dis 2022;14. https://doi.org/10.1177/1759720X221084848. 1759720X221084848.

29. Available at: https://www.fda.gov/drugs/resources-information-approved-drugs/fda-grants-accelerated-approval-infigratinib-metastatic-cholangiocarcinoma#:~:text=On%20May%2028%2C%202021%2C%20theF. Accessed June 25, 2023.

30. Komla-Ebri D, Dambroise E, Kramer I, et al. Tyrosine kinase inhibitor NVP-BGJ398 functionally improves FGFR3-related dwarfism in mouse model. J Clin Invest 2016;126(5):1871–84.

31. Available at: https://investor.bridgebio.com/news-releases/news-release-details/bridgebio-pharma-announces-positive-interim-results-phase-2. Accessed June 25, 2023.

32. Garcia S, Dirat B, Tognacci T, et al. Postnatal soluble FGFR3 therapy rescues achondroplasia symptoms and restores bone growth in mice. Sci Transl Med 2013;5(203):203ra124.

33. Available at: https://clinicaltrials.gov/ct2/show/NCT04638153. Accessed June 25, 2023.

34. Matsushita M, Hasegawa S, Kitoh H, et al. Meclozine promotes longitudinal skeletal growth in transgenic mice with achondroplasia carrying a gain-of-function mutation in the FGFR3 gene. Endocrinology 2015;156(2):548–54.

35. Matsushita M, Esaki R, Mishima K, et al. Clinical dosage of meclozine promotes longitudinal bone growth, bone volume, and trabecular bone quality in transgenic mice with achondroplasia. Sci Rep 2017;7(1):7371.

36. Kitoh H, Matsushita M, Mishima K, et al. Pharmacokinetics and safety after once and twice a day doses of meclizine hydrochloride administered to children with achondroplasia. PLoS One 2020;15(4):e0229639.

37. Kimura T, Bosakova M, Nonaka Y, et al. An RNA aptamer restores defective bone growth in FGFR3-related skeletal dysplasia in mice. Sci Transl Med 2021;13(592). https://doi.org/10.1126/scitranslmed.aba4226.

38. Available at: https://www.ribomic.com/eng/pipeline/rbm007.php. Accessed June 25, 2023.

39. Wrobel W, Pach E, Ben-Skowronek I. Advantages and disadvantages of different treatment methods in achondroplasia: a review. Int J Mol Sci 2021;22(11). https://doi.org/10.3390/ijms22115573.

40. Available at: https://clinicaltrials.gov/ct2/show/NCT04219007?term=selected+genetic+causes+of+short+stature&draw=2&rank=1. Accessed June 25, 2023.

Spinal Muscular Atrophy
A (Now) Treatable Neurodegenerative Disease

Alex Fay, MD, PhD*

KEYWORDS

- Spinal muscular atrophy • Gene therapy • Motor neuron disease
- Newborn screening

KEY POINTS

- Spinal muscular atrophy is an autosomal recessive motor neuron disease that causes progressive weakness, and the infantile-onset type I disease is fatal if untreated in infants.
- Three recently approved treatments are available to treat SMA, and can lead to profound improvements in the natural history of disease, especially in younger patients.
- More rare subtypes of SMA may manifest with unique patterns of muscle weakness, and are best identified through next-generation sequencing panels, whole-exome, or whole-genome sequencing panels.

Spinal muscular atrophy (SMA) is an autosomal recessive disease of the motor neurons, beginning most commonly in infancy, with a wide range of severity, whose devastating natural history has been altered in recent years by the availability of three FDA-approved treatments: nusinersen, onasemnogene abeparvovec, and risdiplam. These novel treatments take advantage of the unique genetics of SMA, and together with newborn screening programs in most states, offer a chance to treat many children in the pre-symptomatic phase of the disease, preventing both death and disability. In this article, I will review the clinical presentation, genetics, and treatment landscape for SMA, and the implications for SMA and related disorders.

HISTORY

The first description of SMA appeared in the 1890s, with case reports by Guido Werdnig (Graz, Austria, 1891),[1] Johan Hoffmann (Heidelberg, Germany, 1893, 1897),[2] and Thomsen and Bruce (Edinburgh, Scotland, 1893).[3] Although the severe form of type I SMA, carries the eponym Werdnig-Hoffmann, the cases described by these two physicians are more consistent with type 2 SMA. Charles Beevor (London, 1903)[4] provided the first description of the severe (type 1) variant of SMA in a family where four children died by 6 months of age, with Jonathan Hutchison (London, 2010),[5]

University of California, San Francisco, 1875 4th Street., Suite 5A, San Francisco, CA 94158, USA
* Corresponding author.
E-mail address: Alexander.fay@ucsf.edu

Pediatr Clin N Am 70 (2023) 963–977
https://doi.org/10.1016/j.pcl.2023.06.002
0031-3955/23/© 2023 Elsevier Inc. All rights reserved.

pediatric.theclinics.com

providing more detailed descriptions of this fatal form. Eric Kugelberg and Lisa Welander (Sweden)[6] together described a milder form with adolescent onset in 1956, and type 3 SMA carries the eponym Kugelberg-Welander disease. Kugelberg and Welander noted that the clinical presentation was similar to limb-girdle muscular dystrophy, but given the neurogenic features in muscle, suggested that this might be a more severe form of Werdnig-Hoffmann disease. Victor Dubovitz (London)[7] wrote the first series describing the intermediate form, type 2 SMA, including 12 children who achieved independent sitting, but not standing, in 1964, and this form carries the eponym Dubovitz disease.

The genetics of SMA was elucidated in 1990 by Gilliam[8] and Melki,[9] who independently identified the chromosome 5q locus, and demonstrated that both the milder and more severe forms mapped to this locus. Melki and colleagues then reported the sequencing of the survival motor neuron gene (SMN) gene at this locus, which is duplicated with the active *SMN1* gene and the mostly inactive *SMN2* gene. The number of copies of *SMN2* would later be found to correlate with disease severity, though it is not the only determinant.

CLINICAL

Although SMA is most often divided into three subtypes, type 1 (onset prior to 6 months, no independent sitting achieved), type 2 (onset 6–18 months, sitting achieved, but not standing) and type 3 (independent standing and walking achieved, but be lost subsequently), a type 0 and type 4 have been described at the extremes, with the fetal onset and adult onset, respectively (**Table 1**). I will describe each of these forms in more detail later in discussion.

SMA manifests with proximal weakness, typically sparing the facial muscles, except in the most severe neonatal cases, though infants with type 1 SMA will develop facial

Table 1
Subtypes of spinal muscular atrophy

SMA Subtype	Age of Onset	Motor Milestones	Life Expectancy (Untreated)	Other Features
0	Antenatal/Birth	Never Sit Independently	<3 months	Contractures Early respiratory failure Facial diplegia
1	<6 months	Never Sit Independently	<2 years	Hypotonia Tongue fasciculations Frog leg posture Face spared early Bell-shaped chest Respiratory failure Tube feeding
2	6–18 months	Sit, Never Stand/Walk	~70% alive at 25 years	Hypotonia Proximal weakness Scoliosis Restrictive Lung Disease Hand tremor
3	18 months-17 years	Walk Independently	Normal	Proximal weakness Hand tremor May Lose Ambulation
4	>18 years	Normal Early Motor Development	Normal	Proximal weakness Hand tremor

weakness as the disease progresses. Given the proximal weakness pattern, SMA may appear to have a similar presentation to congenital myopathies and muscular dystrophies. In the past, electrodiagnostic studies, including electromyography and nerve conduction studies, and muscle biopsy were used routinely for diagnosis. However, with the availability of free or relatively low-cost genetic testing for SMA and muscle diseases, more invasive testing is not usually necessary.

Type 0

This most severe form was reported in a case series by MacLeod and colleagues in 1999,[10] where they described 5 cases of children with reduced fetal movements, severe hypotonia, areflexia, and minimal movements at birth, with death within the first three months of life. Some had multiple contractures (arthrogryposis), bell-shaped chest and tongue fasciculations, and all were confirmed to have loss of both copies of exons 7 and 8 in the SMN1 gene. Two of these patients had absent sensory nerve action potentials, and pathologic analysis in one showed loss of sensory axons within the spinal cord (with extensive abnormalities in subcortical structures, brainstem, cerebellum, and the anterior horn cells), and in another, axon loss in the sural nerve.

One child with type 0 SMA who was treated with nusinersen was reported to have died from cardiac arrest at 5 months of age.[11] This rare, but severe subtype is also providing motivation for fetal intervention in antenatally diagnosed cases of SMA.[12]

Type 1

This most common form of SMA accounts for approximately 60% of cases, with symptoms manifesting after birth, but prior to 6 months, with no achievement of independent sitting. Weakness of proximal muscles is present at the time of diagnosis, while facial muscle movement and distal limb movements are preserved early in the disease course; with disease progression, all muscles are eventually affected. Prior to the availability of targeted treatments, survival beyond two years of age without permanent ventilation and gastrostomy tube was unusual, though some individuals with milder symptoms achieved some head control.[13] Scores of motor function, measured with the CHOP-INTEND scale and other metrics, do not improve in type I SMA.[14,15] Respiratory dysfunction is primarily due to weakness of the intercostal muscles, with relative sparing of the diaphragm[16]; this pattern leads to loss of rib cage volume and the bell-shaped chest observed in infants with type 1 SMA, as well as a reduced ratio of alveoli to bronchi/bronchioles.[17] Nasogastric or gastrostomy tube feeding is typically necessary around 8 months of age.[18] Cognitive impairment is reported in some small series of patients with type I SMA,[19] in line with pathological studies showing abnormalities in the thalamus and other parts of the brain.[20]

Type 2

Although less rapidly degenerative than type 1, type 2 SMA can still be life-limiting, due to progressive scoliosis and restrictive lung disease, though most patients survive to adulthood,[21] with a study in 1997 showing 68.5% survival at 25 years of age.[22] Natural history studies have combined patients with type 2 and type 3 disease, but the children with type 2 SMA can be distinguished by their age of onset being between 6 and 18 months of age and their achievement of independent sitting, but not independent standing or walking. Scoliosis, contractures, and polyminimyoclonus of the hands are common findings. Motor scores, such as the Expanded Hammersmith Functional Motor Scale (HFMSE), correlate with the amplitude of motor nerve compound action potentials (CMAP), as well as with SMN2 copy number. Motor function and forced vital capacity decline slowly, compared to type 1 SMA, and in a non-linear fashion. A more recent natural history study[23] demonstrates some of the challenges in studying therapeutic interventions, as motor scores, upper limb function, and forced vital capacity show distinct trends over 12- 24 months: for example, MFM scores decreased significantly over 24 months, but not over 12 months, while %FVC decline decreased over 12 months but not 24 months, and upper limb strength decreased at 12 and 24 months. Baseline %FVC is higher in individuals with type 3 compared those with type 2, and declines at a slower rate.[24,25]

Type 3

Children with this form of SMA have normal lifespan and achieve ambulation, typically between one and four years of age.[26] This category of SMA has been divided into type IIIA (onset before 3 years of age) and type IIIB (onset after 3 years of age). Ambulatory children with SMA typically show improvements in gait until 6 years of age, at which point there is a slow decline until puberty, followed by a more rapid decline until 20 years of age, and then a slowed rate of decline in adulthood.[27] The declines in ambulation are likely due primarily to weight gain during puberty, while scoliosis and respiratory dysfunction are uncommon. A Polish study[28] showed that the probability of loss of ambulation SMA3 was 80% after a disease duration of 10 years, 68% after 20 years, and 61% after 30 years. Upper extremity strength and respiratory function do decline over time, particularly after the loss of ambulation.[29]

Type 4

This mildest subtype of SMA is also the least common, making up fewer than 5% of SMA cases.[14] Lifespan is normal, and acquisition of motor milestones is normal in childhood, with the onset of proximal weakness and fatigue in adulthood. Ambulation may be preserved throughout life, but if lost, this typically occurs after 50 years of age. Tongue fasciculations and polyminimyoclonus of the fingers can be seen in some individuals. The mean age at diagnosis in a Dutch cohort was 40 years old.[30]

GENETICS

The unique genetics of SMA derives from a duplication of several genes on the long arm of chromosome 5 (5q), creating two highly homologous genes, SMN1 and SMN2. SMA is caused by the loss of both copies of SMN1, a gene which produces fully functional SMN protein. SMN2, by virtue of several nucleotide differences compared to SMN1, leads to the exclusion of exon 7 in 90% of transcripts, creating an unstable protein product and consequently lower level of expression of SMN protein (**Fig. 1A**). The most important of these is the c.840C>T mutation that creates an exonic splicing suppressor site in exon 7, leading to its removal during splicing.

Lack of exon 7 leads to a truncated protein product that is degraded. In a patient with SMA, there is a complete reliance on the SMN2 genes for the expression of SMN protein, and so, in general, more copies of SMN2 provides more SMN protein and a milder phenotype. Most individuals have 2-3 copies of SMN2, leading to a phenotype of type 1, type 2, or type 3 SMA, while at the extremes, 1 copy leads to type 0 and 4-5 copies typically leads to a mild type 3 or type 4 phenotype.

Although 95% of SMA cases are due to the deletion of both copies of SMN1, dozens of point mutations, including nonsense, missense, frameshift, and splice-site mutations, account for the other 5%, with a range of reported phenotypic severity.[31]

Several genetic modifiers within the SMN2 gene and in other genes, have been reported to influence the clinical phenotype of SMA, beyond SMN2 copy number. A point mutation in SMN2 in exon 7, c.859G>C, for example, can increase exon 7

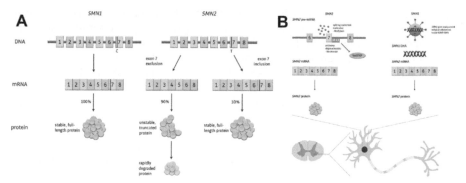

Fig. 1. Genetics of Spinal Muscular Atrophy (*A*). Mechanisms of approved therapies for SMA, showing splicing correction by nusinersen and risdiplam, and SMN gene replacement using adeno-associated virus (AAV) vector (*B*). *Credit*: Maya Dhar.

incorporation and render the phenotype less severe.[32] Deletions of other genes near the *SMN1* locus, particularly *NAIP*, are often associated with a more severe phenotype.[33] There are several families with individuals who have loss of both copies of *SMN1*, and yet have no motor neuron disease. Genetic studies of these families have led to the discovery of several genes that seem to compensate for the loss of *SMN1*, including the actin-binding protein plastin-3.[34] In mice and in cell lines, overexpression of plastin-3 or one of its binding proteins, the actin-binding CORO1C, both of which are important for endocytosis, can rescue endocytosis defects in SMN-depleted cells lines and neuronal defects in animal models of SMA.[35] Another study found a deletion in the neurocalcin delta gene in non-disease-manifesting individuals with loss of both copies of *SMN1*. Knockdown of neurocalcin delta rescues endocytosis defects in SMA cells lines and rescues several aspects of the SMA phenotype in mouse, zebrafish, and worm models of SMA.[36] Other modifier genes identified similarly include neuritin-1 (elevated),[37] an SMN-interacting protein involved in neurite outgrowth and TLL-2 (reduced),[38] an inhibitor of myostatin, a blocker of muscle growth. Interestingly, myostatin inhibitors, which can promote muscle hypertrophy, are under investigation as therapeutics for SMA.[39] Epigenetic factors, too, have been implicated in *SMN2* expression, due to the differential methylation of CpG islands within the *SMN2* promotor,[40] findings which prompted trials exploring the effects of HDAC inhibitor valproic acid on SMA.[41] While results were promising in mice,[42] only a subpopulation of patients seems to benefit, and trial results were disappointing.[43,44]

SMN protein is expressed ubiquitously and plays a role in assembling the small heteronuclear ribonucleoproteins that are part of the spliceosome, as well as in RNA axonal transport. It is not well understood why motor neurons are particularly vulnerable to loss of SMN protein, though rare reports of severely affected infants with symptoms in other tissues suggest that the phenotype may be broader than motor neuron disease: there are reports of cardiac defects,[45] vascular anomalies,[46] abnormalities of the sensory neurons[47] and thalamic neurons,[20] increased pancreatic β-cell islets[48] and disordered fatty acid metabolism.[49]

PREVIOUS TRIALS

Prior to the last 6 years, where several targeted treatments have transformed the management of SMA, many small molecules were investigated as disease modifiers.

These include valproic acid and phenylbutyrate, HDAC inhibitors, as mentioned above, and albuterol, creatine, hydroxyurea, olesoxime, thyrotropin-releasing hormone, and somatotropin. Albuterol (salbutamol) at a dose of 2 mg three times daily demonstrated modest benefits in maintaining motor function[50] and respiratory function among children with type 2 SMA.[51] This may be related to the dysfunction of the neuromuscular junction[52] and to direct effects on increasing SMN2 transcripts and SMN protein levels.[53] Olesoxime is a cholesterol-related compound that protects mitochondria from oxidative damage, and while initial studies suggested a stabilization of motor function in children with type 2 and 3 SMA, longer follow up did not show a benefit.[54] Studies of phenylbutyrate,[55] riluzole,[56] hydroxyurea,[57] creatine, gabapentin, and somatotropin, among other treatments, failed to show benefit in small trials.[58]

Targeted Therapies: Nusinersen, Onasemnogene Abeparvovec, Risdiplam

Nusinersen

A dramatic shift in the SMA treatment landscape began in 2016 with the first disease-modifying drug approval by the US Food and Drug Association (FDA), for nusinersen. This approval was the culmination of decades of work to uncover the unique genetics of SMA, development of animal models of SMA, and using antisense oligonucleotide technology to modify the splicing of SMN2 to increase the incorporation of exon 7 (**Fig. 1**B). The first trial, ENDEAR, was performed in infants with symptomatic type 1 SMA, randomized to sham or intrathecal delivery of the antisense oligonucleotide with four loading doses, followed by continued dosing every 4 months. The results were dramatic, showing increased survival (defined as survival without permanent ventilation), improvement of motor functional scores, and acquisition of milestones not seen in type 1 SMA.[59,60] FDA approval across all age groups and all subtypes of SMA was based on this trial, as well as a small cohort of older patients with SMA types 2 and 3. Notably, earlier treatment (<3 months) was associated with more robust response, whereas children treated at 5 months or beyond generally showed less improvement. A subsequent open-label trial in presymptomatic infants, NURTURE, showed even more dramatic improvements, with none of the participants requiring permanent ventilation, all sitting independently, and 88% walking independently.[61] A subsequent trial in later onset type 2 and 3 SMA showed modest, but steady benefits in motor function, upper limb strength, and acquisition of motor milestones, including independent ambulation in some children, while sham-treated patients showed decline or no improvement in motor function.[62] Side effects of nusinersen have generally been mild, and primarily related to lumbar puncture, and include headache, back pain, and pyrexia.

Onasemnogene abeparvovec

Gene therapy for SMA, onasemnogene abeparvovec, was approved by the FDA in 2019 after results of a trial of infants with symptomatic type I SMA showed increased survival and improved motor function compared to a natural history control group.[63,64] The gene therapy vector is based on adeno-associated virus (AAV) subtype 9, with a CMV enhancer and chicken ß-actin promoter to allow for ubiquitous expression, and is delivered as a single intravenous dose. FDA approval was granted for children under 24 months of age, regardless of SMN2 copy number. As with nusinersen, treatment of symptomatic infants beyond 5 months of age was associated with less robust treatment response,[65] though children beyond 7 months of age appear to tolerate gene therapy and make motor progress.[66] Pre-symptomatic treatment of infants with two or three copies of SMN2 leads to the achievement of normal Bayley motor scores in all infants with three copies of SMN2[67] and in a majority of infants with two copies of SMN2.[68] Treatment response is sustained for at least 6 years, with long-term follow up of the first patients to receive gene therapy.[69] All children are treated with corticosteroids for one day prior to, and at least 30 days after gene therapy infusion, to limit allergic and other inflammatory responses (primarily affecting the liver and heart), and prior to treatment, children must have low levels of anti-AAV antibodies to limit chances of an immune response against the vector and transfected cells. Early side effects include fever, nausea, and vomiting, as well as increases in transaminases and/or troponin-I, and thrombotic microangiopathy (TMA). Nausea and vomiting can be treated with fluids (oral or intravenous) and anti-emetics, while transaminitis and elevated troponin-I are treated by increasing the steroid dose. TMA is treated with supportive care, though in some cases, plasma exchange or anti-complement therapy is necessary. Recent reports of two children with fatal liver disease following gene therapy, during taper of steroids, add another layer of caution in considering this therapy.[70]

Risdiplam

The first oral medication for SMA, risdiplam, was approved in 2020, on the basis of early results from two trials, FIREFISH and SUNFISH, and requires once daily dosing. Risdiplam is a small molecule modifier of splicing, which, such as nusinersen, promotes the inclusion of exon 7 into SMN2 transcripts. FIREFISH[71] included infants with symptomatic type 1 SMA, ages 1-7 months of age, and demonstrated improvements in survival without permanent ventilation, motor developmental milestone acquisition, and independent feeding compared to historical controls, with overall similar results to nusinersen and onasemnogene abeparvovec. In contrast to the earlier studies of nusinersen and onasemnogene abeparvovec, the placebo-controlled SUNFISH[72] trial explored treatment effects in a broad range of non-ambulatory children and young adults, ages 2-25 years of age. Results demonstrated improvements in motor function using the MFM32 and RULM scales, whereas changes in respiratory function were not statistically significant. Based on data from these trials, the FDA approved risdiplam in children older than two months of age and adults. There is an ongoing trial for presymptomatic infants, RAINBOWFISH, but results have not yet been published. Although there was a concern for retinal toxicity in non-human primates treated with risdiplam, this side effect has not been observed in human trials, thus far.[73] The most common adverse events are fever, pneumonia, upper respiratory tract infection, diarrhea, oral ulcers, rash, urinary tract infections, and joint pain.

The costs of each these novel therapies for SMA are enormous, as shown in **Table 2**, as much as $2.125 million for a single dose of onasemnogene abeparvovec, and yearly costs in the hundreds of thousands of dollars for nusinersen and risdiplam. With the expansion of newborn screening to include SMA, infants can be treated in the pre-symptomatic period, where maximum benefit is anticipated. Comparative studies among the three treatments are lacking, and differences in study populations and outcome measures make direct comparisons challenging.[74] Although there are scattered reports of patients treated with a combination of therapies (usually gene therapy, followed by risdiplam or nusinersen), it is not yet clear that there is an additive effect of dual therapy. A trial (NCT04488133) is underway to explore the benefits of nusinersen following gene therapy, using an open-label design, and a similar study will be needed for risdiplam to assess the impact of combined therapy. Cost-effectiveness has been explored in several studies,[75–77] with differing results depending on the model used and the health care system; longer-term follow-up of treated patients will likely help to clarify the cumulative benefits of each therapy.

Table 2
Approved therapies for spinal muscular atrophy

Therapy	Type of Drug	Delivery Route	Frequency	Ages (USA)	Cost
Nusinersen	Antisense Oligonucleotide	Intrathecal	Every 4 Months	All	$750K first year, then $375K/yr
Onasemnogene abeparvovec	Gene Therapy	Intravenous	Single Dose	0–24 months	$2.125 M
Risdiplam	Small molecule	Oral	Daily	>2 months	$100K–$340K/yr

Box 1
Spinal muscular atrophies beyond chromosome 5q

Dominant
  Distal or lower extremity-predominant
    TRPV4 (HMN8, may also cause scapuloperoneal weakness)
    DYNC1H1 (SMA-LED1, CMT2O)
    BICD2 (SMA-LED2)
    HSPB1 (HMN2B, CMT2F; may also be recessive)
    HSPB3 (HMN2C)
    HSPB8 (HMN2A, CMT2L)
    AARS (CMT2N)
    GARS (HMN5A, CMT2D)
    HARS (HMN5A)
    WARS (dHMN9)
    REEP1 (HMN5B)
    BSCL2 (HMN5C)
    SLC5A7 (HMN7A; with vocal cord paralysis)
    DCTN1 (HMN7B; with vocal cord paralysis)
    SETX (with upper motor neuron findings)
    KCC3/SLC12A6 (Andermann syndrome)
    SPTAN1
    MME
    SLC5A6
    COQ7
    HINT1
    TBCK
    FBXO38 (calf-predominant)
    FBLN5 (with macular disease)
    MYH14 (with hearing loss)
    GBF1
  Proximal
    VAPB (ALS8)
    CHCHD10 (SMAJ, FTD-ALS2)
    MORC2 (CMT2Z)
    TFG (CMT2G)
    MAPT (allelic with frontotemporal dementia)

Recessive
  Proximal
    SMA with Respiratory Distress
    IGHMBP2 (SMARD1)
    SMA with congenital bone fractures
    TRIP4
    ASCC1
    SMA with Pontocerebellar hypoplasia
    VRK1 (PCH1A)
    EXOSC3 (PCH1B)
    SMA with Myoclonic Epilepsy
    ASAH1
    SMA with Encephalopathy
    TBCD
  Distal
    PLEKHG5
    DNAJB2 (AR- CMT2)
    REEP1
    SIGMAR1
    SYT2
    SORD (AR-CMT2)

X-linked
  Proximal
    UBE1
  Distal
    ATP7A
    AIFM1
    LAS1L (SMARD2)
Mitochondrial
  mtDNA
    mtATP6
    mtATP8
  Nuclear DNA
    CHCHD10 (SMAJ)
    DGUOK
    SCO2
    SLC25A21
    TK2

Categories of Non-5q SMA Listed by Pattern of Weakness (Proximal or Distal), Mode of Inheritance, and Other Special Features.

Although the three approved treatments are potentially curative when given presymptomatically, children and adults treated beyond the neonatal period have ongoing weakness, even if disease progression is slowed or halted. Thus, additional strategies to improve motor outcomes are needed as adjunctive therapies to the current gene therapy, nusinersen, and risdiplam. The treatment horizon for SMA includes trials of combination therapies, intrathecal gene therapy (NCT05089656), fetal treatment[12] and addition of myostatin inhibitors to currently approved medications. Myostatin is an inhibitor of muscle growth, and inhibitors have been explored as monotherapy in muscular dystrophies, without significant benefit.[78,79] However, ongoing trials (NCT03921528, NCT05115110) aim to determine whether myostatin inhibitors can promote additional growth and strength following or concurrent with the approved SMA therapies. Higher doses of nusinersen are also being explored in patients previously treated with risdiplam (NCT05067790).

Non-5q spinal muscular atrophy

Beyond SMN1-related SMA, there are dozens of genes that can lead to various subtypes of spinal muscular atrophy and hereditary motor neuropathies,[80] many with distinguishing features beyond motor neurons, and some with emerging therapies. Many of these genes overlap with Charcot-Marie-Tooth disease, hereditary spastic paraplegia, mitochondrial disorders, and disorders with combined central and peripheral nervous system dysfunction, such as pontocerebellar hypoplasia and myoclonic epilepsy. The term "hereditary motor neuropathy (HMN)" is interchangeable with "spinal muscular atrophy," as both terms refer to the dysfunction of the peripheral motor neurons. **Box 1** summarizes the non-5q SMA subtypes. One subtype of note from a therapeutic perspective is SMA with respiratory distress, type 1 (SMARD1), which is associated with recessive mutations in the *IGHMBP2* gene.[81] This form of SMA often manifests with sudden respiratory decline in infancy, which can be fatal, superimposed on a phenotype of hypotonia with distal-predominant weakness. Based on promising results in a mouse model of SMARD1,[82] a gene therapy trial is now underway to treat patients with SMARD1 and the allelic, later-onset Charcot-Marie-Tooth disease, type 2S (NCT05152823).

SUMMARY

The last 6 years have brought transformative changes to the treatment of SMA, with three approved therapies that are lifesaving in the infantile period and life-altering across the age spectrum. Newborn screening will allow for the greatest benefit of each therapy, as treatment can be started in the pre-symptomatic period. Still, many patients will continue to have residual motor disability, so adjunctive therapies, combined therapies, and improved delivery of current treatments to motor neurons will be needed. The achievements in treating this neurodegenerative disease offer hope for other, more rare forms of SMA, and for neurological diseases across the lifespan.

CLINICS CARE POINTS

- Spinal muscular atrophy should be suspected in infants and toddlers with hypotonia and weakness of proximal muscle groups in the arms and legs
- Spinal muscular in older children and adults may manifest similarly to limb-girdle muscular dystrophy, and should be considered in the differential diagnosis of patients with proximal muscle weakness and elevated creatine kinase
- Intravenous gene replacement therapy is available for children under 2 years of age in the USA (under 20 kg in the EU)
- Oral and intrathecal drugs that modify the splicing of the SMN2 transcript are can prevent disease progression across the age spectrum
- Treatment should be started as soon as possible after diagnosis to preserve motor neuron function and to prevent the progression of weakness

DISCLOSURES

Consulting for Sarepta, Aeglea, Retrotope, Ultragenyx; Research funding from Sarepta, United States, Elenae; Data Safety Monitoring Board for Aspiro.

REFERENCES

1. Werdnig G. Zwei frühinfantile hereditäre Fälle von progressiver Muskelatrophie unter dem Bilde der Dystrophie, aber auf neurotischer Grundlage. Archiv fur Psychiatrie und Nervenkrankheiten, Berlin 1891;22:437–81.
2. Hoffmann J. Über chronische spinale Muskelatrophie im Kindesalter auf familiärer Basis. Deut Zeitsch Nervenheilkd 1893;3:427–70.
3. Thomson J, Bruce A. Progressive muscular atrophy in a child with a spinal lesion. Edinb Hosp Rep 1893;1:372.
4. Beevor CE. A case of congenital spinal muscular atrophy (family type) and a case of hemorrhage into the spinal cord at birth, giving similar symptoms. Brain 1902; 25:85–108.
5. Hutchinson R. Lectures on diseases of children. 2nd ed. London: Edward Arnold; 1910. p. 276. Fig. 32 (plate).
6. Kugelberg E, Welander L. Heredofamilial juvenile muscular atrophy simulating muscular dystrophy. AMA Arch Neurol Psychiatry 1956;75(5):500–9.
7. Dubowitz V. Infantile muscular atrophy. A prospective study with particular reference to a slowly progressive variety. Brain 1964;87:707–18.

8. Gilliam TC, Brzustowicz LM, Castilla LH, et al. Genetic homogeneity between acute and chronic forms of spinal muscular atrophy. Nature 1990;345:823–5.

9. Melki J, Abdelhak S, Sheth P, et al. Gene for chronic proximal spinal muscular atrophies maps to chromosome 5q. Nature 1990;344:767–8.

10. MacLeod MJ, Taylor JE, Lunt PW, et al. Prenatal onset spinal muscular atrophy. Eur J Paediatr Neurol 1999;3(2):65–72.

11. Tiberi E, Costa S, Pane M, et al. Nusinersen in type 0 spinal muscular atrophy: should we treat? Ann Clin Transl Neurol 2020;7(12):2481–3.

12. Schwab ME, Shao S, Zhang L, et al. Investigating attitudes toward prenatal diagnosis and fetal therapy for spinal muscular atrophy. Prenat Diagn 2022;42(11): 1409–19.

13. Pane M, Palermo C, Messina S, et al. An observational study of functional abilities in infants, children, and adults with type 1 SMA. Neurology 2018;91(8):e696–703.

14. Kolb SJ, Coffey CS, Yankey JW, et al. Natural history of infantile-onset spinal muscular atrophy. Ann Neurol 2017;82(6):883–91.

15. Mercuri E, Lucibello S, Perulli M, et al. Longitudinal natural history of type I spinal muscular atrophy: a critical review. Orphanet J Rare Dis 2020;15(1):84.

16. Kuzuhara S, Chou SM. Preservation of the phrenic motoneurons in Werdnig-Hoffmann disease. Ann Neurol 1981;9:506–10.

17. Cunningham M, Stocks J. Werdnig-Hoffmann disease. The effects of intrauterine onset on lung growth. Arch Dis Child 1978;53:921–5.

18. Finkel RS, McDermott MP, Kaufmann P, et al. Observational study of spinal muscular atrophy type I and implications for clinical trials. Neurology 2014;83: 810–7.

19. Masson R, Brusa C, Scoto M, et al. Brain, cognition, and language development in spinal muscular atrophy type 1: a scoping review. Dev Med Child Neurol 2021; 63(5):527–36.

20. Shishikura K, Hara M, Sasaki Y, et al. A neuropathologic study of Werdnig-Hoffmann disease with special reference to the thalamus and posterior roots. Acta Neuropathol 1983;60(1–2):99–106.

21. Chung BH, Wong VC, Ip P. Spinal muscular atrophy: survival pattern and functional status. Pediatrics 2004;114(5):e548–53.

22. Zerres K, Rudnik-Schoneborn S, Forrest E, et al. A collaborative study on the natural history of childhood and juvenile onset proximal spinal muscular atrophy (type II and III SMA): 569 patients. J Neurol Sci 1997;146:67–72.

23. Chabanon A, Seferian AM, Daron A, et al. Prospective and longitudinal natural history study of patients with Type 2 and 3 spinal muscular atrophy: Baseline data NatHis-SMA study. PLoS One 2018;13(7):e0201004.

24. Souchon F, Simard LR, Lebrun S, et al. Clinical and genetic study of chronic (types II and III) childhood onset spinal muscular atrophy. Neuromuscul Disord 1996;6(6):419–24.

25. Kaufmann P, McDermott MP, Darras BT, et al. Prospective cohort study of spinal muscular atrophy types 2 and 3. Neurology 2012;79(18):1889–97.

26. Kaneko K, Arakawa R, Urano M, et al. Relationships between long-term observations of motor milestones and genotype analysis results in childhood-onset Japanese spinal muscular atrophy patients. Brain Dev 2017;39(9):763–73.

27. Montes J, McDermott MP, Mirek E, et al. Ambulatory function in spinal muscular atrophy: age-related patterns of progression. PLoS One 2018;13(6):e0199657.

28. Lusakowska A, Jedrzejowska M, Kaminska A, et al. Observation of the natural course of type 3 spinal muscular atrophy: data from the polish registry of spinal muscular atrophy. Orphanet J Rare Dis 2021;16(1):150.

29. Wolfe A, Scoto M, Milev E, et al. Longitudinal changes in respiratory and upper limb function in a pediatric type III spinal muscular atrophy cohort after loss of ambulation. Muscle Nerve 2021;64(5):545–51.

30. Wadman RI, Stam M, Gijzen M, et al. Association of motor milestones, SMN2 copy and outcome in spinal muscular atrophy types 0-4. J Neurol Neurosurg Psychiatry 2017;88:365–7.

31. Butchbach MR. Genomic variability in the survival motor neuron genes (SMN1 and SMN2): implications for spinal muscular atrophy phenotype and therapeutics development. Int J Mol Sci 2021;22(15):7896.

32. Prior TW, Krainer AR, Hua Y, et al. A positive modifier of spinal muscular atrophy in the SMN2 gene. Am J Hum Genet 2009;85(3):408–13.

33. Burlet P, Burglen L, Clermont O, et al. Large scale deletions of the 5q13 region are specific to Werdnig-Hoffmann disease. J Med Genet 1996;33:281–3.

34. Oprea GE, Kröber S, McWhorter ML, et al. Plastin 3 is a protective modifier of autosomal recessive spinal muscular atrophy. Science 2008;320(5875):524–7.

35. Hosseinibarkooie S, Peters M, Torres-Benito L, et al. The power of human protective modifiers: PLS3 and CORO1C unravel impaired endocytosis in spinal muscular atrophy and rescue SMA phenotype. Am J Hum Genet 2016;99(3): 647–65.

36. Riessland M, Kaczmarek A, Schneider S, et al. Neurocalcin delta suppression protects against spinal muscular atrophy in humans and across species by restoring impaired endocytosis. Am J Hum Genet 2017;100(2):297–315.

37. Yener IH, Topaloglu H, Erdem-Ozdamar S, et al. Transcript levels of plastin3 and neuritin1 modifer genes in spinal muscular atrophy siblings. Pediatr Int 2017; 59:53–6.

38. Jiang J, Huang J, Gu J, et al. Genomic analysis of a spinal muscular atrophy (SMA) discordant family identifies a novel mutation in TLL2, an activator of growth differentiation factor 8 (myostatin): a case report. BMC Med Genet 2019;20(1):204.

39. Barrett D, Bilic S, Chyung Y, et al. A randomized phase 1 safety, pharmacokinetic and pharmacodynamic study of the novel myostatin inhibitor apitegromab (SRK-015): a potential treatment for spinal muscular atrophy. Adv Ther 2021;38(6): 3203–22.

40. Hauke J, Riessland M, Lunke S, et al. Survival motor neuron gene 2 silencing by DNA methylation correlates with spinal muscular atrophy disease severity and can be bypassed by histone deacetylase inhibition. Hum Mol Genet 2009; 18(2):304–17.

41. Sumner CJ, Huynh TN, Markowitz JA, et al. Valproic acid increases SMN levels in spinal muscular atrophy patient cells. Ann Neurol 2003;54(5):647–54.

42. Tsai LK, Tsai MS, Ting CH, et al. Multiple therapeutic effects of valproic acid in spinal muscular atrophy model mice. J Mol Med (Berl) 2008;86(11):1243–54.

43. Swoboda KJ, Scott CB, Crawford TO, et al. SMA CARNI-VAL trial part I: double-blind, randomized, placebo-controlled trial of L-carnitine and valproic acid in spinal muscular atrophy. PLoS One 2010;5(8):e12140.

44. Kissel JT, Scott CB, Reyna SP, et al. SMA CARNIVAL TRIAL PART II: a prospective, single-armed trial of L-carnitine and valproic acid in ambulatory children with spinal muscular atrophy. PLoS One 2011;6(7):e21296.

45. Rudnik-Schöneborn S, Heller R, Berg C, et al. Congenital heart disease is a feature of severe infantile spinal muscular atrophy. J Med Genet 2008;45(10): 635–8.

46. Araujo Ap, Araujo M, Swoboda KJ. Vascular perfusion abnormalities in infants with spinal muscular atrophy. J Pediatr 2009;155(2):292–4.

47. Rudnik-Schoneborn S, Goebel HH, Schlote W, et al. Classical infantile spinal muscular atrophy with SMN deficiency causes sensory neuronopathy. Neurology 2003;60:983–7.

48. Bowerman M, Swoboda KJ, Michalski JP, et al. Glucose metabolism and pancreatic defects in spinal muscular atrophy. Ann Neurol 2012;72(2):256–68.

49. Crawford TO, Sladky JT, Hurko O, et al. Abnormal fatty acid metabolism in childhood spinal muscular atrophy. Ann Neurol 1999;45(3):337–43.

50. Frongia AL, Natera-de Benito D, Ortez C, et al. Salbutamol tolerability and efficacy in patients with spinal muscular atrophy type II. Neuromuscul Disord 2019;29(7):517–24.

51. Khirani S, Dabaj I, Amaddeo A, et al. Effect of salbutamol on respiratory muscle strength in spinal muscular atrophy. Pediatr Neurol 2017;73:78–87.e1.

52. Pera MC, Luigetti M, Sivo S, et al. Does albuterol have an effect on neuromuscular junction dysfunction in spinal muscular atrophy? Neuromuscul Disord 2018; 28(10):863–4.

53. Angelozzi C, Borgo F, Tiziano FD, et al. Salbutamol increases SMN mRNA and protein levels in spinal muscular atrophy cells. J Med Genet 2008;45(1):29–31.

54. Muntoni F, Bertini E, Comi G, et al. Long-term follow-up of patients with type 2 and non-ambulant type 3 spinal muscular atrophy (SMA) treated with olesoxime in the OLEOS trial. Neuromuscul Disord 2020;30(12):959–69.

55. Mercuri E, Bertini E, Messina S, et al. Randomized, double-blind, placebo-controlled trial of phenylbutyrate in spinal muscular atrophy. Neurology 2007; 68(1):51–5.

56. Russman BS, Iannaccone ST, Samaha FJ. A phase 1 trial of riluzole in spinal muscular atrophy. Arch Neurol 2003;60(11):1601–3.

57. Chen TH, Chang JG, Yang YH, et al. Randomized, double-blind, placebo-controlled trial of hydroxyurea in spinal muscular atrophy. Neurology 2010;75(24):2190–7.

58. Wadman RI, van der Pol WL, Bosboom WM, et al. Drug treatment for spinal muscular atrophy types II and III. Cochrane Database Syst Rev 2020;1(1):CD006282.

59. Finkel RS, Mercuri E, Darras BT, et al. Nusinersen versus sham control in infantile-onset spinal muscular atrophy. N Engl J Med 2017;377(18):1723–32.

60. Finkel RS, Chiriboga CA, Vajsar J, et al. Treatment of infantile-onset spinal muscular atrophy with nusinersen: a phase 2, open-label, dose-escalation study. Lancet 2016;388(10063):3017–26.

61. De Vivo DC, Bertini E, Swoboda KJ, et al. Nusinersen initiated in infants during the presymptomatic stage of spinal muscular atrophy: Interim efficacy and safety results from the Phase 2 NURTURE study. Neuromuscul Disord 2019;29(11): 842–56.

62. Mercuri E, Darras BT, Chiriboga CA, et al. Nusinersen versus sham control in later-onset spinal muscular atrophy. N Engl J Med 2018;378(7):625–35.

63. Mendell JR, Al-Zaidy S, Shell R, et al. Single-dose gene-replacement therapy for spinal muscular atrophy. N Engl J Med 2017;377(18):1713–22.

64. Day JW, Finkel RS, Chiriboga CA, et al. Onasemnogene abeparvovec gene therapy for symptomatic infantile-onset spinal muscular atrophy in patients with two copies of SMN2 (STR1VE): an open-label, single-arm, multicentre, phase 3 trial. Lancet Neurol 2021;20(4):284–93.

65. Lowes LP, Alfano LN, Arnold WD, et al. Impact of age and motor function in a phase 1/2A study of infants with SMA type 1 receiving single-dose gene replacement therapy. Pediatr Neurol 2019;98:39–45.

66. Matesanz SE, Battista V, Flickinger J, et al. Clinical experience with gene therapy in older patients with spinal muscular atrophy. Pediatr Neurol 2021;118:1–5.

67. Strauss KA, Farrar MA, Muntoni F, et al. Onasemnogene abeparvovec for pre-symptomatic infants with three copies of SMN2 at risk for spinal muscular atrophy: the Phase III SPR1NT trial. Nat Med 2022;28(7):1390–7.

68. Strauss KA, Farrar MA, Muntoni F, et al. Onasemnogene abeparvovec for pre-symptomatic infants with two copies of SMN2 at risk for spinal muscular atrophy type 1: the Phase III SPR1NT trial. Nat Med 2022;28(7):1381–9.

69. Mendell JR, Al-Zaidy SA, Lehman KJ, et al. Five-year extension results of the phase 1 START trial of onasemnogene abeparvovec in spinal muscular atrophy. JAMA Neurol 2021;78(7):834–41.

70. Available at: https://www.reuters.com/business/healthcare-pharmaceuticals/novartis-reports-zolgensma-caused-two-deaths-liver-failure-2022-08-11/. September 18, 2022.

71. Darras BT, Masson R, Mazurkiewicz-Bełdzińska M, et al. Risdiplam-treated infants with type 1 spinal muscular atrophy versus historical controls. N Engl J Med 2021;385(5):427–35.

72. Mercuri E, Deconinck N, Mazzone ES, et al. Safety and efficacy of once-daily risdiplam in type 2 and non-ambulant type 3 spinal muscular atrophy (SUNFISH part 2): a phase 3, double-blind, randomised, placebo-controlled trial. Lancet Neurol 2022;21(1):42–52.

73. Sergott RC, Amorelli GM, Baranello G, et al. Risdiplam treatment has not led to retinal toxicity in patients with spinal muscular atrophy. Ann Clin Transl Neurol 2021;8(1):54–65.

74. Erdos J, Wild C. Mid- and long-term (at least 12 months) follow-up of patients with spinal muscular atrophy (SMA) treated with nusinersen, onasemnogene abeparvovec, risdiplam or combination therapies: a systematic review of real-world study data. Eur J Paediatr Neurol 2022;39:1–10.

75. Dean R, Jensen I, Cyr P, et al. An updated cost-utility model for onasemnogene abeparvovec (Zolgensma®) in spinal muscular atrophy type 1 patients and comparison with evaluation by the institute for clinical and effectiveness review (ICER). J Mark Access Health Policy 2021;9(1):1889841.

76. Broekhoff TF, Sweegers CCG, Krijkamp EM, et al. Early cost-effectiveness of onasemnogene abeparvovec-xioi (zolgensma) and nusinersen (spinraza) treatment for spinal muscular atrophy I in the netherlands with relapse scenarios. Value Health 2021;24(6):759–69.

77. Zuluaga-Sanchez S, Teynor M, Knight C, et al. Cost effectiveness of nusinersen in the treatment of patients with infantile-onset and later-onset spinal muscular atrophy in Sweden. Pharmacoeconomics 2019;37(6):845–65.

78. Campbell C, McMillan HJ, Mah JK, et al. Myostatin inhibitor ACE-031 treatment of ambulatory boys with Duchenne muscular dystrophy: Results of a randomized, placebo-controlled clinical trial. Muscle Nerve 2017;55(4):458–64.

79. Leung DG, Bocchieri AE, Ahlawat S, et al. A phase Ib/IIa, open-label, multiple ascending-dose trial of domagrozumab in fukutin-related protein limb-girdle muscular dystrophy. Muscle Nerve 2021;64(2):172–9.

80. Available at: https://neuromuscular.wustl.edu/synmot.html. Accessed September 20, 2022.

81. Eckart M, Guenther UP, Idkowiak J, et al. The natural course of infantile spinal muscular atrophy with respiratory distress type 1 (SMARD1). Pediatrics 2012; 129(1):e148–56.

82. Nizzardo M, Simone C, Rizzo F, et al. Gene therapy rescues disease phenotype in a spinal muscular atrophy with respiratory distress type 1 (SMARD1) mouse model. Sci Adv 2015;1(2):e1500078.

Recognizing and Managing a Metabolic Crisis

Peter R. Baker II, MD

KEYWORDS

- Inborn error of metabolism • Hyperammonemia • Metabolic acidosis • Anion gap
- Lactate • Ketone • Catabolism • Sodium phenylbutyrate

KEY POINTS

- Metabolic emergencies can occur at any age, are gender non-specific, and if not recognized and treated can result in permanent disability or death.
- Basic laboratories including blood gas, comprehensive metabolic panel, urine/plasma ketones, and plasma lactate and ammonia can facilitate recognition at most medical centers.
- Acute treatment includes providing calories (typically with dextrose) and detoxification (with dialysis and some disease-specific therapies).
- Vitamin and nutritional interventions for specific disorders are useful in acute treatment, as well as chronic management to avoid future metabolic emergencies.

INTRODUCTION

Inborn errors of metabolism (IEM) are genetic disorders involving biochemical pathways throughout the body. Categorically, there are subsets of these disorders that cause acute intoxication, energy deficiency, and acidosis, resulting in a clinical metabolic emergency.[1] These conditions include urea cycle disorders (UCD), organic acidemias (OA), maple syrup urine disease (MSUD), fatty acid oxidation disorders (FAOD), and primary lactic acidosis (PLA). There is great overlap in clinical presentation with these disorders.[2] They are characterized by an asymptomatic period (one day to many years), followed by the onset of symptoms including vomiting, poor feeding (particularly in neonates), lethargy, irritability, hallucinations, slurred speech, rapid breathing, seizures, loss of consciousness, coma, and eventually death.[3] These symptoms, as a broad group, are called symptoms of intoxication. In the absence of known exogenous intoxicant ingestion, these symptoms should prompt the clinician to consider an IEM in the differential diagnosis.[1]

University of Colorado, Children's Hospital Colorado, 13123 East 16th Avenue, Box 300, Aurora, CO 80045, USA
E-mail address: Peter.Bakerli@CUAnschutz.edu

Pediatr Clin N Am 70 (2023) 979–993
https://doi.org/10.1016/j.pcl.2023.05.009
0031-3955/23/© 2023 Elsevier Inc. All rights reserved.

pediatric.theclinics.com

The onset of a metabolic emergency is precipitated by "metabolic stress." This can be due to an overwhelming amount of substrate in a blocked metabolic pathway (eg, too much oral protein intake in a UCD). More commonly onset is precipitated by catabolism, or the body's mobilization of its own nutrients/substrates, for energy. Catabolism can be caused by fasting (not eating/drinking calories), vomiting in the setting of an infectious illness (losing calories), inadequate caloric intake for needs (not eating/drinking *enough* calories during times of increased caloric needs), or deficit of specific nutrients for prolonged periods of time (eg, withholding protein for days).[2,4] In these settings, the body naturally releases its own internal energy stores of fatty acids (from adipose) and amino acids (typically from muscle), which can overwhelm blocked pathways and result in the buildup of toxic metabolites. Simultaneously, because of the primary metabolic block, the cell may not be able to produce enough energy further resulting in cellular damage and/or death.[5]

Episodes of metabolic stress and crisis can recur throughout the lifetime of the individual.[6-11] Whether it is exogenous substrate overload or endogenous catabolism that cause the metabolic emergency, recognizing the crisis and treating in a timely manner can be the difference between an individual living without disease sequelae or suffering life-altering end-organ damage. During crisis, in all of these disorders, the central nervous system can suffer permanent damage to the cortex, white matter, and/or basal ganglia, leading to irreversible sequelae including dystonia, epilepsy, spasticity, paralysis, and/or intellectual disability (depending on which areas of the brain are damaged). MSUD uniquely can present with a sweet odor (particularly in the ear wax, and eventually in urine). MSUD is one of the few disorders that has a progressive prodrome of apnea, opisthotonos, and reflexive "bicycling" movements in the first days of life.[12] Other organs beyond the central nervous system can be affected as well. The liver can be damaged in UCD, OA, and FAOD.[13] Cardiomyopathy or rhabdomyolysis can be a presenting symptom in FAOD, particularly long-chain disorders.[11] In the most severe settings delayed treatment in any of these disorders can lead to death.

Through current newborn screening, many of these conditions (but not all) can be detected and managed within the first week of life. Sometimes, due to the severity of the condition, diagnosis by newborn screen can come *after* the onset of symptoms (day of life 2 or 3). In such cases, or in conditions that are missed by newborn screening, a high index of suspicion needs to be maintained. This is especially true in the neonatal intensive care unit, but holds true through every stage of life from the pediatric clinic and emergency medicine, to internal medicine, obstetrics, and the adult intensive care unit.[6-11]

Diagnosis of these IEM is accomplished through several mechanisms. Newborn screen will detect many disorders and prompt further work-up. In disorders not screened, patients may present symptomatically. In either case biochemical testing of blood and urine, genetic testing, and enzymatic testing are helpful in diagnostic confirmation. Once a diagnosis is confirmed, management can be targeted to the specific disease, and often includes diet modification, avoidance of fasting, vitamin and nutritional supplements, and intervention to prevent an acute metabolic crisis from occurring.

This article will outline easy and basic steps to detect, or at least raise suspicion for, a metabolic emergency using basic laboratory tests available in most health care facilities. It details specialty testing that can be sent to support a metabolic diagnosis. Finally, it discusses easy, rapid interventions that can mitigate damage and reverse metabolic intoxication during an acute event.

Basic Laboratory Studies to Detect a Metabolic Crisis

While genetic testing is useful to confirm a diagnosis, it is not typically the first step in diagnosing an IEM. If the individual has symptoms of intoxication there are several laboratory studies that are available in almost any health care setting, and useful in providing clues toward a diagnosis. **Fig. 1** describes symptoms of intoxication, basic initial laboratories to obtain, interpretation of these lab results in the most common disorders, and next steps in metabolic work-up.

The most basic and often obtained study is the "comprehensive metabolic panel." Several elements can be helpful in a metabolic emergency. Plasma bicarbonate, combined with venous or arterial blood gas, is useful in an acute intoxication event. In UCD including ornithine transcarbamylase deficiency (OTC) and Citrullinemia Type 1 there is a respiratory alkalosis.[5] In other metabolic emergencies, anion gap metabolic acidosis is detectable using these basic labs. Using plasma chloride, sodium, and bicarbonate anion gap metabolic acidosis[5] is seen in OA and PLA, due to over production of ketones and/or lactate. In FAOD there may also be elevated in lactate due to the secondary inhibition of pyruvate carboxylase. Elevations in either lactate or plasma ketones resulting in anion gap metabolic acidosis are not unique to IEM, but can be used as non-specific markers. Lactate is commonly elevated in severe infection/sepsis, tissue necrosis, cardiac malformations, and in the setting of poor tissue perfusion. In evaluating for these other conditions, considering an IEM would be appropriate.

In a neonate, regardless of blood glucose, ketones should not be elevated to the point of being detectable in the urine, or high enough to cause anion gap acidosis.[14,15] While ketones are produced in neonates, and are important for supplying energy to the central nervous system, elevation of urine ketones (easily detected using a bedside urine dipstick or laboratory-based urinalysis) in a neonate (particularly in the first week of life) is strongly suggestive of an OA.[5,9]

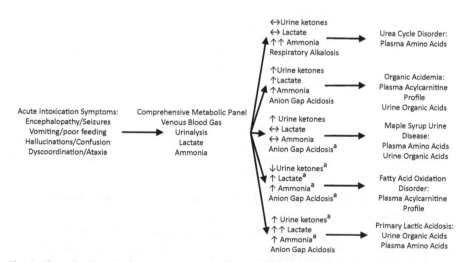

Fig. 1. Flow diagram describing the interpretation of basic, widely available laboratory findings in the setting of a metabolic emergency. The presence of symptoms of acute intoxication should prompt obtaining these labs. Findings should prompt further investigation using specialty biochemical labs to aid in the diagnosis of the inborn error of metabolism.
[a]Variable based on age and/or severity.

In a non-neonatal healthy individual, ketones should be elevated in the setting of low blood glucose and/or prolonged fasting, and result in anion gap metabolic acidosis. This is termed physiologic ketosis and is necessary for the brain and heart to operate in starvation. A lack of elevation (hypoketosis) during fasting and hypoglycemia may indicate a FAOD.[5] Blood glucose can be, but is not always, low in acutely presenting IEM.[5] Particularly profound (blood glucose <20 mg/dL) or refractory hypoglycemia can be indicative of a metabolic disorder.

Elevated transaminases (alanine aminotransferase and aspartate aminotransferase) are markers of hepatocellular damage. This can be present in FAOD, OA, UCD, and PLA.[5] Hepatic synthetic dysfunction (evident by elevated low albumin and high INR) may be present. This degree of hepatic dysfunction can be seen particularly in UCD and FAOD.[5] Combined hepatopathy and encephalopathy (Reye-like presentation) should raise concern for an intoxicating IEM as well.[16] In long-chain FAOD, elevations in transaminases may also originate from the muscle and be a sign of rhabdomyolysis.[17] In this case, creatinine kinase (CK) would be elevated as well.

One final and relatively ubiquitous laboratory analysis is plasma ammonia. Hyperammonemia is one of the primary intoxicating metabolites in most IEM with an acute phenotype, including in UCD, OA, FAOD, and even in some PLA.[5] Whether it is the primary driver of intoxication in all of these disorders is controversial and confounded by energy deficits to vital organs such as the brain and liver, metabolic acidosis, and derangement of other bioactive compounds including organic and amino acids. High plasma ammonia (>60–100 μM) should raise concern for an IEM, especially in the setting of intoxication symptoms and the other aforementioned laboratory abnormalities. There are many other etiologies of hyperammonemia including primary liver failure/insufficiency, vascular malformations, toxin or drug exposure, neoplasm, and urease-producing infection, to name a few. Care should be taken to investigate such etiologies concomitantly with IEM.

There are several other caveats regarding hyperammonemia. First, in a neonate, normal ammonia can be up to 100 to 125 μM. In older children and adults, these levels would be considered moderately elevated, so keeping the age of the patient in mind is important. Although most laboratories report ammonia in units of "micromol/L" (micromolar, μM), some laboratories use μg/dL. With a conversion factor of ~0.6 from μg/dL to micromol/L (eg, 170 μg/dL = 100 μM) care should be taken to clarify units and reference range when considering whether an individual is hyperammonemic. Finally, and very importantly, blood ammonia levels can be falsely elevated and dependent on how a sample is drawn and handled. If it is drawn with a tourniquet, drawn under strain or pressure, sampled by heal/capillary blood, allowed to sit at room temperature, or allowed to sit for prolonged period before processing in the lab, elevated values should be viewed with caution.[18] Ammonia should be drawn through a free-flowing line, without a tourniquet, placed on ice immediately, and processed in the lab as soon as possible (ideally within 30–40 minutes).

Specialty Laboratories and Diagnostic Confirmation of an Intoxicating Inborn Errors of Metabolism

Specialty biochemical tests are processed and interpreted in a Clinical Biochemical Laboratory. Most health care centers around the United States do not have a Clinical Biochemical Laboratory available on site. Most clinicians send samples to a regional academic or commercial center, usually once a biochemical genetics specialist is involved. Still, understanding what types of tests are sent to and processed by such laboratories, and their utility in diagnosing intoxicating IEM is important in understanding the overall evaluation for the presence of an IEM. Unless there is a laboratory that can process these samples on-site, real-time decision-making based on results during an acute metabolic crisis is not possible. Results that return in 24 to 48 hours may have some utility in acute management, but largely these tests are sent to support diagnostic testing rather than to guide treatment. They are also used in some cases to optimize nutritional management in the more chronic, outpatient clinical setting.

There are 3 main specialty biochemical tests that are ordered when assessing for the etiology of acute metabolic crisis: plasma amino acids, urine organic acids, and plasma acylcarnitines, also known as the plasma acylcarnitine profile. Plasma amino acids can help in the evaluation of UCD, OA, MSUD, and PLA. In UCD glutamine is elevated as a result of hyperammonemia; alanine and/or glycine may be elevated as well.[19] Depending on the type of UCD other amino acids are variably affected. Citrulline is low in proximal UCD such as OTC Deficiency, and it is elevated in distal UCD including Citrullinemia Type 1[19]. Citrulline may also be elevated in the PLA, pyruvate carboxylase deficiency. Arginine can be high (Arginase Deficiency) or low (Citrullinemia Type 1) depending on which enzyme in the urea cycle is affected.[19] The amino acid pattern alone may be diagnostic of a UCD. In OA, amino acids are not specific for any single condition, but generally glycine is high and glutamine is low compared to the reference range.[9,20] In MSUD, the branched chain amino acids leucine, isoleucine, and valine are elevated, as well as the pathognomonic elevation of alloisoleucine.[21] Finally, alanine is typically elevated in chronic lactic acidosis, and thus can be useful in diagnosing PLA.[22]

Urine organic acids are helpful in diagnosing most of these metabolic conditions. The primary use of UOA is in diagnosing and distinguishing types of OA. Specific patterns will be present for methylmalonic acidemia (MMA), propionic acidemia (PA), and isovaleric acidemia (IVA) that are diagnostic for each condition.[23] MSUD has variable elevations in alpha-ketoacids, as well as ketones (acetoacetate and beta-hydroxybutyrate).[12] FAO may have non-specific elevations in dicarboxylic acids. In MCAD deficiency the presence of hexanoylglycine can be diagnostic. UCD (specifically OTC deficiency) will have orotic acid and uracil that is detectable in a UOA sample.[9] PLA, as expected, demonstrates elevated lactate, but plasma concentrations are typically higher (above 6–10 mM), and more refractory to treatment than other etiologies.

Finally, the plasma acylcarnitine profile is useful in detecting OA and FAOD. In OA, there will be elevations of C3 (propionylcarnitine) acylcarnitine for MMA and PA, and C5 (isovalerylcarnitine) in IVA.[24] Specific acylcarnitine patterns can be seen in, and are diagnostic for medium-chain (C8, octanoylcarnitine), very long-chain (C14:1, myristoylcarnitine), and long-chain hydroxy (C16-OH, hydroxy-palmitoylcarnitine) acyl-coA dehydrogenase deficiencies. Carnitine Palmitoyl Transferase type 1 (CPT1) typically has high free carnitine and low long-chain species (eg, C18, stearoylcarnitine), while Carnitine Acylcarnitine Translocase (CACT) deficiency and Carnitine Palmitoyl Transferase type 2 (CPT2) deficiency have low free carnitine and elevated long-chain species (eg, C18).[24] Ketone-related acylcarnitines (C2, acetylcarnitine and C4-OH, hydroxy-butyrylcarnitine) are low in these disorders.

Besides biochemical testing, the confirmation of an IEM, and potentially understanding the severity, requires molecular testing (gene sequencing) and/or enzymatic testing. Alternatively, the use of genomic sequencing including rapid whole exome, or rapid/ultra-rapid whole genome sequencing, can achieve a diagnosis within days, and is now often preferred over single gene and panel testing that may take weeks. The former can be obtained using blood, saliva, or buccal swab, and there are many commercial laboratories that offer single gene or gene panel testing. The decision regarding what test to get is guided by biochemical pattern and clinical features. Enzymatic testing is more rarely done. It often requires skin fibroblasts obtained from a biopsy. Some studies are optimized for leukocytes, which is less invasive. Due to maintenance cost, disease rarity, and improved molecular testing, many enzymatic assays are no longer clinically available.

TREATMENT OF METABOLIC CRISIS: STOP THE PRECURSOR, REVERSE CATABOLISM, AND START DETOXIFICATION

There are 3 major principles to the general treatment of a metabolic crisis/emergency. The application of these principles to each categorical disorder can be found in **Table 1**. First, any offending precursors need to be stopped. In UCD, OA, and MSUD, this is protein. In FAOD it is fat, however it is not clear whether this is acutely harmful.[25] In emergency fluid management FAOD are the only group of conditions in which lipids should be withheld for caloric repletion. Of note, in UCD and OA protein should not be held for too long (no longer than 24 hours), because withholding protein alone can induce protein catabolism of muscle. After ~24 hours a small amount of protein (eg, 0.8 mg/kg/d (d)) should be reintroduced enterally or parenterally.[26] In MSUD parenteral amino acid mixtures free of leucine are used.[27]

Second, because the emergency is typically being triggered by metabolic stress which induces catabolism, catabolism must be stopped. As above, catabolism occurs with prolonged fasting, vomiting, and/or infection. Often these all occur at once. In some instances, catabolism can be triggered by a medication such as steroids. To reverse/treat catabolism, dextrose with appropriate electrolytes should be administered. Typically, D10 in normal saline given at 1.5 times the maintenance rate is used. This provides roughly 8 to 10 gm/kg/min glucose.[26] It is important to maintain relatively high glucose infusion rates. If blood glucose begins to climb (>80–110 mg/dL), it is preferable to not lower the GIR, but rather to begin insulin to facilitate intracellular transport of glucose.[26] Intralipid can be added to the anabolic regimen if the patient does not have a FAOD. Typically, 2-3 g/kg/d of 20% lipid emulsion is sufficient.[26] In adults we may only use 1 g/kg/d based on tolerance and dietary needs. Very rarely are dextrose or lipids contraindicated. Lipids should theoretically not be given in FAOD. In PLA-like pyruvate dehydrogenase (PDH) deficiency, excess dextrose can exacerbate lactic acidosis by overwhelming glycolysis, therefore a ~4:1 lipid-to-carbohydrate ratio parenteral nutrition has been suggested.[26] Chronically, use of a ketogenic diet may be beneficial. Generally, the use of less dextrose and more lipid is less effective in other PLA such as mitochondrial respiratory chain disorders. Here, adequate caloric support with a careful balance of dextrose and lipid is optimal.[26] Dextrose is contraindicated in Citrullinemia Type II, where protein and lipids are the preferred regimen, and dextrose can exacerbate a hyperammonemic crisis.[28]

Finally, when possible, detoxification should be started to decrease levels of the intoxicating chemical. Typically, this is ammonia, but may also be organic acids and/or lactate. In UCD sodium phenylbutyrate and sodium benzoate can be used in hyperammonemia.[29–31] These ammonia "scavengers" bind glutamine and glycine to generate phenylacetyl glutamate and hippuric acid, respectively. These chemicals can be excreted in urine. As the major reservoirs of ammonia in the blood, binding glutamine and glycine is a highly effective way of bringing the bodies circulating ammonia levels down.[31] They are administered with arginine.[9,32] Any of these can be given enterally through a gastric or nasogastric tube.[29] Ideally, however, these are given intravenously using the formulation Ammonul.[31] Use of this drug may be limited by cost and/or availability.

Arguably, Ammonul should not be used in OA.[30] While the sodium benzoate component could be effective to lower glycine (which is often elevated), there is not an

Table 1
Disorders that can cause a metabolic emergency/crisis (and some examples of these disorders), followed by the primary clinical features, specialty biochemical testing, and management points

Disorder	Examples	Main Clinical Features	Primary Biochemical Test	Primary Treatments	Vitamins/Supplements
Urea Cycle	N-Acetylglutamate Synthase (NAGS) Deficiency Ornithine Transcarbamylase (OTC) Deficiency Citrullinemia Type 1	Respiratory alkylosis Hyperammonemia Liver dysfunction	Plasma Amino Acids	Dextrose, Lipid Withhold/reduce Protein Ammonia Scavengers Carglumic acid Hemodialysis	Arginine or citrulline in OTC deficiency
Organic Acidemias	Methylmalonic Acidemia (MMA) Propionic Acidemia (PA) Isovaleric Acidemia (IVA)	Anion gap metaoblic acidosis Ketoacidosis Lactic acidosis Hyperammonemia Liver dysfunction	Urine Organic Acids Plasma Acylcarnitine Profile	Dextrose, Lipid Withhold/reduce Protein Carglumic Acid Hemodialysis	Levocarnitine Hydroxocobalamin (some forms of MMA) Glycine(IVA) Biotin (some forms of PA)
Amino Acidopathy	Maple Syrup Urine Disease (MSUD)	Ketoacidosis Sweet odor (ear wax) Spasticity, bicycling, opisthotonos	Plasma Amino Acids Urine Organic Acids	Dextrose, Lipid Withhold/reduce Protein Leucine Supplement Isoleucine and Valine Hemodialysis	Isoleucine and valine supplmentation Thaimine (some forms of MSUD)
Fatty acid oxidation	Medium-Chain Acyl-CoA Dehydrogenase (MCAD) Deficiency Multiple Acyl-CoA Dehydrogenase Deficiency (MADD) Long-Chain Disorders Very Long Chain Acyl-CoA Dehydrogenase	Anion gap metaoblic acidosis Hypoketotic Hypoglycemia Lactic acidosis Hyperammonemia Liver dysfunction Cardiomyopathy (LC only)	Plasma Acylcarnitine Profile	Dextrose	Levocarnitine used in MCADD and MADD Low doses and with caution in VLCADD Triheptanoin used in long chain disorders

(continued on next page)

Table 1
(continued)

Disorder	Examples	Main Clinical Features	Primary Biochemical Test	Primary Treatments	Vitamins/Supplements
	(VLCAD) Deficiency Carnitine-Acyl-Carnitine Translocase (CACT) Deficiency Carnitine Palitoyl Transferase Type 2 (CPT2) Deficiency Long Chain Hydroxy Acyl-CoA Dehdrogenase (LCHAD) Deficiency	Rhabdomyolysis (LC only)			
Primary lactic acidosis	Pyruvate Dehydrogenase (PDH) Deficiency Pyruvate Carboxylase (PC) Deficiency Mitochondrial Respiratory Chain Disorders	Anion gap metaoblic acidosis Lactic acidosis Liver dysfunction	Plasma lactate and pyruvate Plasma Amino Acids Urine Organic Acids	Dextrose, Lipid (use of each varies per condition) Hemodialysis	Thiamine (PDH) Ketogenic Diet (PDH)

intravenous form available in the United States. Sodium phenylbutyrate is not typically used in OA mainly because glutamine is not elevated,[9,30] it is low. Giving phenylbutyrate could exacerbate hypoglutaminemia.[33] Further, both components (benzoate and phenylbutyrate) can acidify the mitochondrial matrix, potentially exacerbating dysfunction. A different medication, carglumic acid (N-carbamylglutamate), traditionally used for hyperammonemia in the UCD N-acetylglutamate Synthase (NAGS) Deficiency, is now approved for OA.[29,34–36] The mechanism of hyperammonemia in OA is the inhibition of the synthesis of N-acetylglutamate, a cofactor for the first step in the urea cycle. Carglumic acid replaces the cofactor and allows the urea cycle to function properly.

The most efficient and effective means of detoxification of ammonia in OA, as well as in UCD in which the ammonia is greater than ~300 to 400 micromol/L, is hemodialysis.[37] This is superior to peritoneal dialysis and continuous renal replacement therapy (CRRT),[38] although the latter two therapies could be used if hemodialysis is not possible (particularly due to neonatal size, fragility, access, or on site availability).[39,40] Dialysis is also the preferred means of treating hyperammonemia in acute liver failure. In this setting the enzymes that allow sodium benzoate and sodium phenylbutyrate to work are dysfunctional, rendering these medications much less efficacious. Therefore, the use of them separately or as Ammonul is not proven effective in acute liver failure.[41]

In PLA, FAOD, and OA, lactate, ketones, and some organic acids can contribute to anion gap metabolic acidosis. In most of these disorders, simply reversing catabolism can mitigate the acidosis. Bicarbonate can be used as the blood pH decreases. In severe crises the preferred method of detoxification, as with hyperammonemia, is dialysis.[42,43]

Nutritional Supplements and Cofactors

The principles above broadly cover most IEM in the setting of metabolic crisis. Vitamins and nutritional supplements specific to groups of disorders should be considered to help mitigate metabolic derangements. With a variety of mechanisms (depending on the supplement and the disorder), these can be used in acute crisis situations to regain metabolic control. Frequently they are used on a more chronic basis to maintain control and avoid episodes of crisis in the setting of illness, fasting, or other metabolic stressors.

Levocarnitine is used in treating most OA, both to prevent secondary depletion but also as a detoxifying agent. Particularly, PA, MMA, IVA, and even glutaric acidemia type 1 (GA1, a cerebral organic acidemia) respond well to higher doses of intravenous carnitine (100–400 mg/kg/d) in times of illness.[44–47] In general, carnitine allows for the excretion of toxic organic acid species via conversion from an acyl-CoA molecule (not excretable, trapped within the mitochondria) to an acyl-carnitine molecule (can escape the mitochondria and excretable in urine).[47] Further, the conjugation of an overproduced acyl group (again, usually bound as an acyl-CoA) with carnitine allows the intracellular CoA pool to be available for energy production within the mitochondria.[48] Both mechanisms are thought to mitigate cellular damage in crisis. High doses (>100–200 mg/kg/d) should not be given orally as they could produce adverse effects of gastrointestinal upset, production of trimethylamine, and diarrhea.[49,50] In FAOD, carnitine can be given in medium-chain acyl CoA dehydrogenase deficiency (MCADD) to replete stores depleted by the over-production of medium-chain fatty acyl-CoAs. Some practices will do this only if plasma carnitine levels are low. Some do it empirically in illness. In longer chain disorders (particularly VLCADD) it has been postulated that higher doses of intravenous carnitine are arrhythmogenic. While this is not supported by rigorous study to date, it is a practice cautiously and generally observed in biochemical genetics.

Vitamins can be very helpful in some conditions, in initial crisis-like presentations as well as long term. Hydroxocobalamin (a potent high dose form of vitamin B12) is invaluable in treating inborn errors of cobalamin metabolism that result in elevated MMA and/or homocysteine.[51–54] Subcutaneous hydroxocobalamin, formulated to be given intravenously in the setting of cyanide poisoning in house fires,[55,56] is given daily to reduce MMA and/or homocysteine levels and gain metabolic control, and to maintain lower levels of MMA chronically to avoid/delay onset of chronic renal disease.[52] This form of cobalamin is more efficacious than cyanocobalamin,[57] and it is very safe in the relatively small doses given in cobalamin defects.[54,56] It should be given immediately if there is a suspected OA.[44,52] Some forms of PA and PLA (pyruvate carboxylase deficiency) are responsive to Biotin.[44] Riboflavin (vitamin B2) can be given in the acute management and maintenance management of multiple acyl-CoA dehydrogenase deficiency, and in some rare responsive forms of GA1.[58–61] Thiamin (thiamine; vitamin B1) can be given in some forms of PLA (PDH deficiency) as well as responsive forms of MSUD.[12]

Amino acid supplementation may be given during acute crises, but also chronically for conditions such as IVA (glycine),[47] OTC deficiency (arginine intravenously or oral citrulline),[32] and MSUD (isoleucine and valine).[12] In IVA, glycine is given along with levocarnitine because of its ability to bind with isovaleryl- and 3-hydroxyisovaleryl-CoA, making these excretable and further detoxifying.[47] In OTC deficiency, arginine and/or citrulline act to replenish urea cycle intermediates in crisis. Additionally, citrulline has an added benefit of scavenging extra ammonia into the urea cycle, downstream of the enzymatic block, by incorporating the amine group of aspartate into urea.[32] In MSUD, as leucine is being withheld in acute crises, isoleucine and valine are given to both replete these essential amino acids as well as to help block the transport of cytotoxic leucine across the blood brain barrier, via competition at the LAT1 cation transporter.[62]

In disorders of long-chain fat metabolism, the administration of medium-chain fats (in the form of medium-chain triglycerides, typically composed of 3 molecules of octanoate (C8) on a glycerol backbone) has been used to supplement long-chain fat restriction to treat and prevent acute episodes of rhabdomyolysis as well as subacutely treat cardiomyopathy.[63,64] The efficacy of MCT supplementation has been recently challenged, in favor of a synthetic molecule, triheptanoin. This is a molecule composed of 3 heptanoate (C7) moieties on a glycerol backbone. Using an odd chain fatty acid with both 2- and 3-carbon catabolites, C7 better provides energy to the tricarboxylic acid cycle (TCA) cycle. Head-to-head studies have demonstrated the superiority of triheptanoin for treating cardiomyopathy. It is promising also in the long-term prevention of hospitalizations due to rhabdomyolysis as well.[65,66]

SUMMARY

While individually rare, taken together, metabolic crisis from an IEM is a relatively common phenomenon, which, if not detected and treated immediately, could result in permanent disability or death. An initial/presenting episode can occur in the first few days of life, in the elderly, or anytime in between. Newborn screening has allowed us to detect many, but by no means all, of these conditions before they present acutely. Therefore, a high index of suspicion is required. Suspicion can be easily and quickly substantiated with some basic, widely available labs including urinalysis (ketones), comprehensive metabolic panel, plasma lactate and ammonia, and venous/arterial blood gas. The diagnosis can be confirmed as empiric treatment is being implemented using more sophisticated specialty biochemical labs as well as genetic testing. Safe, empiric treatment includes removing offending substrates, stopping catabolism by giving calories (dextrose and in most cases lipids), and in the setting of hyperammonemia and/or metabolic acidosis, starting a treatment that removes toxins. While there are disease-specific means of doing this, the most effective across nearly all acutely presenting disorders is dialysis. Finally, fine-tuning therapy with supplements of vitamins/cofactors, amino acids, and/or lipid nutritional supplements can be key in maintaining metabolic stability well beyond discharge. Supportive management in illness and avoidance of triggers is important in the chronic management and prevention of metabolic crises across the lifespan.

CLINICS CARE POINTS

- Obatain basic laboratory studies.
- Begin parenteral nutrition (typically glucose to begin).
- Apply specific interventions (vitamins, detoxificants, other nutritional supplements) as labs direct toward a more specific diagnosis.

DISCLOSURE

The author has nothing to disclose.

REFERENCES

1. Saudubray JM, Baumgartner M, Walter J. 6th edition. Inborn metabolic diseases diagnosis and treatment, vol. 1. Berlin: Springer; 2016. p. 658.
2. Saudubray JM, Sedel F, Walter JH. Clinical approach to treatable inborn metabolic diseases: an introduction. J Inherit Metab Dis 2006;29(2–3):261–74.
3. Calvo M, Artuch R, Macia E, et al. Diagnostic approach to inborn errors of metabolism in an emergency unit. Pediatr Emerg Care 2000;16(6):405–8.
4. Takahashi T, Yamada K, Kobayashi H, et al. Metabolic disease in 10 patients with sudden unexpected death in infancy or acute life-threatening events. Pediatr Int 2015;57(3):348–53.
5. Saudubray JM, Garcia-Cazorla A. Inborn Errors of Metabolism Overview: Pathophysiology, Manifestations, Evaluation, and Management. Pediatr Clin North Am 2018;65(2):179–208.
6. Toquet S, Spodenkiewicz M, Douillard C, et al. Adult-onset diagnosis of urea cycle disorders: Results of a French cohort of 71 patients. J Inherit Metab Dis 2021; 44(5):1199–214.
7. Bijvoet GP, van der Sijs-Bos CJ, Wielders JP, et al. Fatal hyperammonaemia due to late-onset ornithine transcarbamylase deficiency. Neth J Med 2016;74(1):36–9.
8. Cavicchi C, Donati M, Parini R, et al. Sudden unexpected fatal encephalopathy in adults with OTC gene mutations-Clues for early diagnosis and timely treatment. Orphanet J Rare Dis 2014;9:105.
9. Kolker S, Garcia-Cazorla A, Valayannopoulos V, et al. The phenotypic spectrum of organic acidurias and urea cycle disorders. Part 1: the initial presentation. J Inherit Metab Dis 2015;38(6):1041–57.

10. Oliveira SF, Pinho L, Rocha H, et al. Rhabdomyolysis as a presenting manifestation of very long-chain acyl-coenzyme a dehydrogenase deficiency. Clin Pract 2013;3(2):e22.

11. Wilcken B. Fatty acid oxidation disorders: outcome and long-term prognosis. J Inherit Metab Dis 2010;33(5):501–6.

12. Strauss KA, Carson VJ, Soltys K, et al. Branched-chain alpha-ketoacid dehydrogenase deficiency (maple syrup urine disease): Treatment, biomarkers, and outcomes. Mol Genet Metab 2020;129(3):193–206.

13. Kolker S, Valayannopoulos V, Burlina AB, et al. The phenotypic spectrum of organic acidurias and urea cycle disorders. Part 2: the evolving clinical phenotype. J Inherit Metab Dis 2015;38(6):1059–74.

14. Sidbury JB Jr, Dong BL. Ketosis in infants and children. J Pediatr 1962;60:294–303.

15. Inokuchi T, Yoshida I, Kaneko A, et al. Neonatal ketosis is not rare: experience of neonatal screening using gas chromatography-mass spectrometry. J Chromatogr B Biomed Sci Appl 2001;758(1):57–60.

16. Goetz V, Yang DD, Lacaille F, et al. What are the clues for an inherited metabolic disorder in Reye syndrome? A single Centre study of 58 children. Mol Genet Metab 2022;135(4):320–6.

17. Weibrecht K, Dayno M, Darling C, et al. Liver aminotransferases are elevated with rhabdomyolysis in the absence of significant liver injury. J Med Toxicol 2010;6(3):294–300.

18. Maranda B, Cousineau J, Allard P, et al. False positives in plasma ammonia measurement and their clinical impact in a pediatric population. Clin Biochem 2007;40(8):531–5.

19. Rodney S, Boneh A. Amino Acid Profiles in Patients with Urea Cycle Disorders at Admission to Hospital due to Metabolic Decompensation. JIMD Rep 2013;9:97–104.

20. Hsia YE, Scully KJ, Rosenberg LE. Inherited propionyl-Coa carboxylase deficiency in "ketotic hyperglycinemia". J Clin Invest 1971;50(1):127–30.

21. Oglesbee D, Sanders KA, Lacey JM, et al. Second-tier test for quantification of alloisoleucine and branched-chain amino acids in dried blood spots to improve newborn screening for maple syrup urine disease (MSUD). Clin Chem 2008;54(3):542–9.

22. Bedoyan JK, Hage R, Shin HK, et al. Utility of specific amino acid ratios in screening for pyruvate dehydrogenase complex deficiencies and other mitochondrial disorders associated with congenital lactic acidosis and newborn screening prospects. JIMD Rep 2020;56(1):70–81.

23. Jones PM, Bennett MJ. Urine organic acid analysis for inherited metabolic disease using gas chromatography-mass spectrometry. Methods Mol Biol 2010;603:423–31.

24. Rinaldo P, Cowan TM, Matern D. Acylcarnitine profile analysis. Genet Med 2008;10(2):151–6.

25. Ficicioglu C, Hussa C. Very long-chain acyl-CoA dehydrogenase deficiency: the effects of accidental fat loading in a patient detected through newborn screening. J Inherit Metab Dis 2009;32(Suppl 1):S187–90.

26. Kripps KA, Baker PR 2nd, Thomas JA, et al. REVIEW: Practical strategies to maintain anabolism by intravenous nutritional management in children with inborn metabolic diseases. Mol Genet Metab 2021;133(3):231–41.

27. Sanchez-Pintos P, Meavilla S, Lopez-Ramos MG, et al. Intravenous branched-chain amino-acid-free solution for the treatment of metabolic decompensation

episodes in Spanish pediatric patients with maple syrup urine disease. Front Pediatr 2022;10:969741.

28. Saheki T, Inoue K, Tushima A, et al. Citrin deficiency and current treatment concepts. Mol Genet Metab 2010;100(Suppl 1):S59–64.

29. Longo N, Diaz GA, Lichter-Konecki U, et al. Glycerol phenylbutyrate efficacy and safety from an open label study in pediatric patients under 2 months of age with urea cycle disorders. Mol Genet Metab 2021;132(1):19–26.

30. Haberle J, Chakrapani A, Ah Mew N, et al. Hyperammonaemia in classic organic acidaemias: a review of the literature and two case histories. Orphanet J Rare Dis 2018;13(1):219.

31. Enns GM, Berry SA, Berry GT, et al. Survival after treatment with phenylacetate and benzoate for urea-cycle disorders. N Engl J Med 2007;356(22):2282–92.

32. Lichter-Konecki U, Caldovic L, Morizono H, et al. Ornithine Transcarbamylase Deficiency. In: Adam MP, Everman DB, Mirzaa GM, et al, editors. GeneReviews. 1993.

33. Filipowicz HR, Ernst SL, Ashurst CL, et al. Metabolic changes associated with hyperammonemia in patients with propionic acidemia. Mol Genet Metab 2006; 88(2):123–30.

34. Valayannopoulos V, Baruteau J, Delgado MB, et al. Carglumic acid enhances rapid ammonia detoxification in classical organic acidurias with a favourable risk-benefit profile: a retrospective observational study. Orphanet J Rare Dis 2016;11:32.

35. Chakrapani A, Valayannopoulos V, Segarra NG, et al. Effect of carglumic acid with or without ammonia scavengers on hyperammonaemia in acute decompensation episodes of organic acidurias. Orphanet J Rare Dis 2018;13(1):97.

36. Burlina A, Bettocchi I, Biasucci G, et al. Long-term use of carglumic acid in methylmalonic aciduria, propionic aciduria and isovaleric aciduria in Italy: a qualitative survey. Eur Rev Med Pharmacol Sci 2022;26(14):5136–43.

37. Eisenstein I, Pollack S, Hadash A, et al. Acute hemodialysis therapy in neonates with inborn errors of metabolism. Pediatr Nephrol 2022. https://doi.org/10.1007/s00467-022-05507-3.

38. Schaefer F, Straube E, Oh J, et al. Dialysis in neonates with inborn errors of metabolism. Nephrol Dial Transplant 1999;14(4):910–8.

39. Celik M, Akdeniz O, Ozgun N, et al. Short-term results of continuous venovenous haemodiafiltration versus peritoneal dialysis in 40 neonates with inborn errors of metabolism. Eur J Pediatr 2019;178(6):829–36.

40. Celik M, Akdeniz O, Ozgun N. Efficacy of peritoneal dialysis in neonates presenting with hyperammonaemia due to urea cycle defects and organic acidaemia. Nephrology 2019;24(3):330–5.

41. De Las Heras J, Aldamiz-Echevarria L, Martinez-Chantar ML, et al. An update on the use of benzoate, phenylacetate and phenylbutyrate ammonia scavengers for interrogating and modifying liver nitrogen metabolism and its implications in urea cycle disorders and liver disease. Expert Opin Drug Metab Toxicol 2017;13(4): 439–48.

42. Vaziri ND, Ness R, Wellikson L, et al. Bicarbonate-buffered peritoneal dialysis. An effective adjunct in the treatment of lactic acidosis. Am J Med 1979;67(3):392–6.

43. Aufricht C, Arbeiter K. Clinical impact of peritoneal equilibration testing in treatment of congenital lactic acidosis by acute peritoneal dialysis. Am J Perinatol 1997;14(3):145–6.

44. Baumgartner MR, Horster F, Dionisi-Vici C, et al. Proposed guidelines for the diagnosis and management of methylmalonic and propionic acidemia. Orphanet J Rare Dis 2014;9:130.
45. Chinen Y, Nakamura S, Tamashiro K, et al. Isovaleric acidemia: Therapeutic response to supplementation with glycine, l-carnitine, or both in combination and a 10-year follow-up case study. Mol Genet Metab Rep 2017;11:2–5.
46. Boy N, Muhlhausen C, Maier EM, et al. Proposed recommendations for diagnosing and managing individuals with glutaric aciduria type I: second revision. J Inherit Metab Dis 2017;40(1):75–101.
47. de Sousa C, Chalmers RA, Stacey TE, et al. The response to L-carnitine and glycine therapy in isovaleric acidaemia. Eur J Pediatr 1986;144(5):451–6.
48. Mitchell GA, Gauthier N, Lesimple A, et al. Hereditary and acquired diseases of acyl-coenzyme A metabolism. Mol Genet Metab 2008;94(1):4–15.
49. Miller MJ, Bostwick BL, Kennedy AD, et al. Chronic Oral L-Carnitine Supplementation Drives Marked Plasma TMAO Elevations in Patients with Organic Acidemias Despite Dietary Meat Restrictions. JIMD Rep 2016;30:39–44.
50. Levocarnitine. Drugs and lactation database (LactMed). https://www.ncbi.nlm.nih.gov/books/NBK501864/.
51. Kripps KA, Sremba L, Larson AA, et al. Methionine synthase deficiency: Variable clinical presentation and benefit of early diagnosis and treatment. J Inherit Metab Dis 2022;45(2):157–68.
52. Huemer M, Diodato D, Schwahn B, et al. Guidelines for diagnosis and management of the cobalamin-related remethylation disorders cblC, cblD, cblE, cblF, cblG, cblJ and MTHFR deficiency. J Inherit Metab Dis 2017;40(1):21–48.
53. Horster F, Tuncel AT, Gleich F, et al. Delineating the clinical spectrum of isolated methylmalonic acidurias: cblA and mut. J Inherit Metab Dis 2021;44(1):193–214.
54. Kacpura A, Frigeni M, Gunther K, et al. Clinical and biochemical outcomes in cobalamin C deficiency with use of high-dose hydroxocobalamin in the early neonatal period. Am J Med Genet 2022;188(6):1831–5.
55. Thompson JP, Marrs TC. Hydroxocobalamin in cyanide poisoning. Clin Toxicol 2012;50(10):875–85.
56. Friedman BT, Chen BC, Latimer AJ, et al. Iatrogenic pediatric hydroxocobalamin overdose. Am J Emerg Med 2019;37(7):1394 e1–e1394 e2.
57. Andersson HC, Shapira E. Biochemical and clinical response to hydroxocobalamin versus cyanocobalamin treatment in patients with methylmalonic acidemia and homocystinuria (cblC). J Pediatr 1998;132(1):121–4.
58. Yildiz Y, Talim B, Haliloglu G, et al. Determinants of Riboflavin Responsiveness in Multiple Acyl-CoA Dehydrogenase Deficiency. Pediatr Neurol 2019;99:69–75.
59. Ribeiro JV, Gomes CM, Henriques BJ. Functional Recovery of a GCDH Variant Associated to Severe Deflavinylation-Molecular Insights into Potential Beneficial Effects of Riboflavin Supplementation in Glutaric Aciduria-Type I Patients. Int J Mol Sci 2020;21(19). https://doi.org/10.3390/ijms21197063.
60. Lucas TG, Henriques BJ, Gomes CM. Conformational analysis of the riboflavin-responsive ETF:QO-p.Pro456Leu variant associated with mild multiple acyl-CoA dehydrogenase deficiency. Biochim Biophys Acta Proteins Proteom 2020;1868(6):140393.
61. Chalmers RA, Bain MD, Zschocke J. Riboflavin-responsive glutaryl CoA dehydrogenase deficiency. Mol Genet Metab 2006;88(1):29–37.
62. Strauss KA, Wardley B, Robinson D, et al. Classical maple syrup urine disease and brain development: principles of management and formula design. Mol Genet Metab 2010;99(4):333–45.

63. Brown-Harrison MC, Nada MA, Sprecher H, et al. Very long chain acyl-CoA dehydrogenase deficiency: successful treatment of acute cardiomyopathy. Biochem Mol Med 1996;58(1):59–65.
64. Ambrose A, Sheehan M, Bahl S, et al. Outcomes of mitochondrial long chain fatty acid oxidation and carnitine defects from a single center metabolic genetics clinic. Orphanet J Rare Dis 2022;17(1):360.
65. Sklirou E, Alodaib AN, Dobrowolski SF, et al. Physiological Perspectives on the Use of Triheptanoin as Anaplerotic Therapy for Long Chain Fatty Acid Oxidation Disorders. Front Genet 2020;11:598760.
66. Gillingham MB, Heitner SB, Martin J, et al. Triheptanoin versus trioctanoin for long-chain fatty acid oxidation disorders: a double blinded, randomized controlled trial. J Inherit Metab Dis 2017;40(6):831–43.

Current Practices in Pharmacogenomics

Laura B. Ramsey, PhD[a,b,c,*], Cynthia A. Prows, MSN, APRN[d],
Sonya Tang Girdwood, MD, PhD[c,e,f], Sara Van Driest, MD, PhD[g]

KEYWORDS

- Pharmacogenetics • Pediatrics • Genomics • Guidelines

KEY POINTS

- Pediatric patients are prescribed medications influenced by pharmacogenomics.
- Guidelines are available for using pharmacogenomics to manage medications in pediatric patients.
- Cases are presented to demonstrate the utility of pharmacogenomics in pediatric patients.

INTRODUCTION

When choosing medications and calculating doses in infants, children, and adolescents, it is common to consider the patient's diagnosis, age, weight, and sometimes body surface area. Despite careful therapeutic decisions, patients may experience inadequate therapeutic effect, a spectrum of adverse effects from mild to severe, or hypersensitivity reactions. Pharmacogenomics (PGx, also referred to as pharmacogenetics), where genomic information is used to tailor medication management, is a strategy to maximize drug efficacy and minimize toxicity. An increasing number of Food and

[a] Division of Clinical Pharmacology, Cincinnati Children's Hospital Medical Center, College of Medicine, University of Cincinnati, 3333 Burnet Avenue, MLC 6018, Cincinnati, OH 45229, USA; [b] Division of Research in Patient Services, Cincinnati Children's Hospital Medical Center, College of Medicine, University of Cincinnati, 3333 Burnet Avenue, MLC 6018, Cincinnati, OH 45229, USA; [c] Department of Pediatrics, University of Cincinnati College of Medicine, 3333 Burnet Avenue, MLC 9016, Cincinnati, OH 45529, USA; [d] Division of Human Genetics, Department of Pediatrics and Center for Professional Excellence, Patient Services, Cincinnati Children's Hospital Medical Center, College of Medicine, University of Cincinnati, 3333 Burnet Avenue, MLC 6018, Cincinnati, OH 45229, USA; [e] Division of Hospital Medicine, Cincinnati Children's Hospital Medical Center, 3333 Burnet Avenue, MLC 9016, Cincinnati, OH 45529, USA; [f] Division of Clinical Pharmacology, Cincinnati Children's Hospital Medical Center, 3333 Burnet Avenue, MLC 9016, Cincinnati, OH 45529, USA; [g] Department of Pediatrics, Vanderbilt University Medical Center, 2200 Children's Way, 8232 DOT, Nashville, TN 37205, USA
* Corresponding author. Division of Clinical Pharmacology, Cincinnati Children's Hospital Medical Center, College of Medicine, University of Cincinnati, 3333 Burnet Avenue, MLC 6018, Cincinnati, OH 45229.
E-mail address: laura.ramsey@cchmc.org

Pediatr Clin N Am 70 (2023) 995–1011
https://doi.org/10.1016/j.pcl.2023.05.010
0031-3955/23/© 2023 Elsevier Inc. All rights reserved.
pediatric.theclinics.com

Drug Administration (FDA) medication labels contain PGx information but do not necessarily recommend or require pre-prescription genetic testing. The Clinical Pharmacogenetics Implementation Consortium (CPIC) is an international group of experts in pharmacology and PGx dedicated to creating expert reviewed, evidence-based, and regularly updated gene-drug clinical practice guidelines.[1] A serial, cross-sectional study that included prescribing information from nearly 2.9 million pediatric patients from 16 sites, reported a conservative annual prescribing prevalence of 8000 to 11,000 per 100,000 patients who received prescriptions for CPIC level A medications (those with prescribing guidelines).[2] However, the systematic implementation of these guidelines to inform medication selection and dosing in pediatrics remains limited.[3]

In some pediatric clinics and hospitals, the implementation of PGx started as early as 2004[4] and has gradually increased.[5] Models for implementation vary between sites.[6] With rising numbers of clinics and hospitals implementing PGx, pediatric providers may encounter past PGx results with therapeutic recommendations for specific medications but are unaware of the applicability of those results to new or additional medications. Patients with complex needs may be exposed to several concurrent medications, and providers may lack knowledge and/or time to consider the evidence for individualized dosing or titration.[3] As other articles in this Special Issue describe, pediatric providers should expect increased use of exome sequencing (ES) and genome sequencing (GS) for diagnostic testing, which will enable opportunistic screening of genes that can influence medication response (pharmacogenes). Only two pharmacogenes (both related to malignant hyperthermia and discussed in Case 3a later in discussion) are currently recommended for opportunistic analysis from ES/GS due to analytical validity concerns for other pharmacogenes.[7]

Pharmacogenes can encode drug-metabolizing enzymes, transporters, drug targets, or immune response proteins. Most well-established pharmacogenes encode drug metabolism enzymes, particularly cytochrome P450 enzymes.[8] The impact of variant pharmacogenes may depend on whether a drug is a pro-drug that is activated by drug-metabolizing enzymes, or an active drug that is metabolized into inactive or active metabolites (**Fig. 1**).

PGx uses a unique nomenclature system that catalogs alleles with star numbers (eg, *1, *2, *3). The *1 allele denotes a "normal" function allele. A star allele can be informed by one or more variants in a gene. The Pharmacogene Variation Consortium (PharmVar) catalogs the star allele nomenclature and functional characterization for many pharmacogenes.[9] The functional consequence of a star allele that codes for a drug-metabolizing enzyme is categorized as: no function, decreased function, normal function, and increased function.[10,11] The phenotype of an individual for each drug-metabolizing enzyme or transporter is determined by the combined functional activity of the maternal and paternal star alleles (called a diplotype). CPIC guidelines include an assessment of the activity of each allele, translation of diplotypes into phenotypes, and dosing recommendations.[1] For genes associated with medication hypersensitivity (eg, *HLA-A, HLA-B*), a single risk allele is associated with hypersensitivity.[10]

To avoid repeating recent reviews in pediatric PGx,[8,12] herein we use a case-based approach to illustrate the use of PGx data in pediatric clinical care. Pharmacogenes featured in cases and their potential phenotypes are in **Table 1**.

CASES AND DISCUSSION
Case 1: Medically Complex Patient

ST is a 9 year-old patient with medical complexity consequent to a non-fatal submersion event resulting in cardiac arrest, anoxic brain injury, severe neurologic impairment,

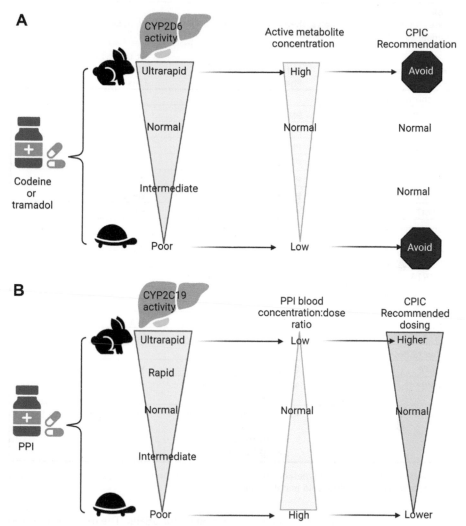

Fig. 1. Examples of a pro-drug being metabolized to an active drug (codeine to morphine, *A*) and active drug being metabolized to an inactive drug (Proton pump inhibitors, (PPIs), *B*) with the blood concentrations and Clinical Pharmacogenetics Implementation Consortium (CPIC) recommendations.[38,44] This figure was created using Biorender.com.

and subsequent need for many medications. She has demonstrated persistent pain and anxiety behaviors attributed to visceral hyperalgesia and likely dysfunction of the neurologic-gut axis, despite formula and medication regimen changes. Parents ask about selective serotonin reuptake inhibitors (SSRIs) and share that they learned from other parents that genetic testing can be used to help manage these medications. *What resources are available to determine if results of PGx testing are relevant for SSRIs?*

Parents are increasingly finding information about PGx testing on the internet and through social networks. Some parents are initiating their child's testing through direct-to-consumer laboratories. Pediatric providers should be prepared to answer parents' questions about PGx testing and to use information from PGx reports.

Table 1
Genes tested in case examples, their potential phenotypes, and the availability of CPIC guidelines

Genes Tested in Case Examples	Potential Reported Phenotypes	At Least 1 Gene-Drug CPIC Published Guideline (Yes/No)
Cytochrome P450 genes:		
CYP2B6	PM, IM, NM, RM, UM	Yes
CYP2C19	PM, IM, NM, RM, UM	Yes
CYP2C9	PM, IM, NM	Yes
CYP2D6	PM, IM, NM, UM	Yes
CYP3A5	PM, IM, NM	Yes
NUDT15	PM, IM, NM	Yes
TPMT	PM, IM, NM	Yes
Transporter genes		
SLC6A4	Normal or low activity	No
Receptor genes		
HTR2A	Normal, intermediate or low activity	No
Hypersensitivity genes		
HLA-A*31:01	Positive, negative	Yes
HLA-B*15:02	Positive, negative	Yes
Other genes		
CFTR	Cystic fibrosis	Yes
RYR1	Malignant hyperthermia susceptibility	Yes
MT-RNR1	MT-RNR1 aminoglycoside-induced hearing loss or nephrotoxicity susceptibility	Yes

Abbreviations: IM, intermediate metabolizer; NM, normal metabolizer; PM, poor metabolizer; RM, rapid metabolizer; UM, ultrarapid metabolizer.

ST's mother specifically asks about genetic testing for SSRIs. The reader is referred to a pragmatic review of considerations whether or not to test[13] and a short, useful guide for pharmacogenetic test selection.[14] Briefly, the first step is to determine if a medication has PGx guidelines or drug label with PGx advice. The Pharmacogenomics Knowledge Database (PharmGKB) is a useful place to start (**Table 2**). Guidelines and recommendations as well as drug labels can be searched with a Pediatric filter (**Fig. 2**). If PGx information is in one or more drug labels, it is tagged as either PGx: testing required, testing recommended, actionable or informative. Specific SSRI guideline recommendations are addressed in Case 2.

Drug-drug interactions must also be considered when a child is on many different medications.[15] Phenoconversion is a type of drug-drug interaction that changes a child's genotype-predicted cytochrome P450 metabolizing phenotype.[15–17] Medications, supplements, or food that act as inducers can increase the activity of a particular drug-metabolizing enzyme, whereas inhibitors can reduce or eliminate enzyme activity (see **Table 2** for resource).

Some pediatric hospitals reduce the burden on clinicians by providing PGx just-in-time information delivery models.[4,6] Consulting with local pharmacists may also be

Table 2
Resources for common questions

Clinical Question	Resources to Find Answers

How do I determine if my patient's PGx test results are relevant for medications I want to prescribe?	Pharmacogenomics Knowledgebase (PharmGKB) Clinical Guideline Annotations[15]
	• Click on Pediatric filter, then search by drug to find related guidelines or recommendations or both with pediatric information published by:
	  ○ The Clinical Pharmacogenetics Implementation Consortium (CPIC)
	  ○ Royal Dutch Association for the Advancement of Pharmacy – Pharmacogenetics Working Group (DPWG)
	  ○ Canadian Pharmacogenomics Network for Drug Safety (CPNDS)
	  ○ French National Network of Pharmacogenetics
	PharmGKB Drug Label Annotations[16]
	• Click on Pediatric filter, then search by drug to determine if PGx information is in a drug label approved by:
	  ○ U.S. Food and Drug Administration (FDA)
	  ○ Health Canada (Sante Canada)
	  ○ European Medicines Agency
	  ○ Swiss Agency of Therapeutic Products
	  ○ Pharmaceuticals and Medical Devices Agency of Japan

How do I find medications that can change a child's genotype-predicted cytochrome P450 metabolizing phenotype?	FDA Drug Development and Drug Interactions Table of Substrates, Inhibitors, and Inducers[17] • Click on "Clinical index inhibitors" or "Clinical index inducers"
How do I find a laboratory that offers PGx testing?	First check with your clinic/hospital's laboratory and use existing service if available. • While a database exists to find laboratories that offer PGx testing, laboratory and test comparison function is not available Consult with local or regional genetic counselor
How do I find a genetic counselor near me?	Use the National Society of Genetic Counselors' search tool: https://findageneticcounselor.nsgc.org/In-Person-FindaGC

helpful as pharmacy practices are increasingly incorporating PGx information into their medication therapy management frameworks.[18] Newer PGx delivery models include genetic counselors, given their expertise in obtaining, evaluating, and communicating genetic test results.[19]

Case 2: Neurology Patient

JP is an 11-year-old nonverbal male with autism spectrum disorder, epilepsy, and worsening aggressive behavior. Current medications are clonidine (for sleep), olanzapine (for agitation), and buspirone (for agitation). In the past, levetiracetam worsened behavior, risperidone caused fatigue and ataxia, and divalproex was ineffective. The patient is admitted to address behavior concerns, where oxcarbazepine and escitalopram are considered. Panel-based PGx testing is done on admission and results are

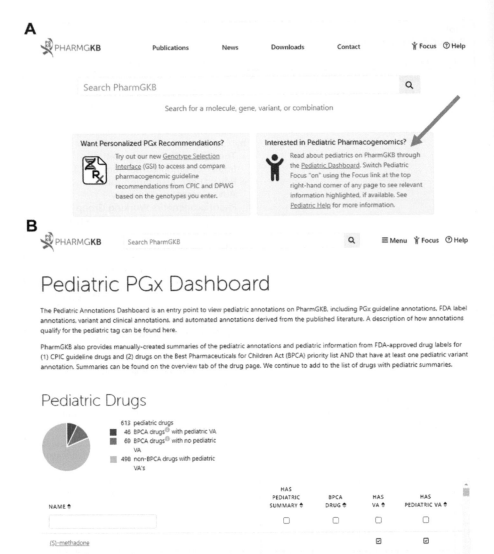

Fig. 2. Find the Pharmacogenomics Knowledgebase (PharmGKB) pediatric website by going to pharmgkb.org and clicking the link for the pediatric website (indicated by the orange *arrow* in *A*) or go straight to what is shown in *panel B* at https://www.pharmgkb.org/pediatric/dashboard.

reflected in **Table 3**. *Which of these results are valuable, and how might they potentially explain prior medication responses and inform future drug choices?*

Panel-based testing may or may not provide results relevant to a patient's current treatment as illustrated in **Table 3**. This patient had panel-based testing for many genes that have no CPIC guidelines relevant to the patient at the time of evaluation, but may be useful in the future (eg, if this patient were prescribed NSAIDs the CYP2C9 result would be relevant).[20] There are CPIC guidelines for oxcarbazepine[21] and escitalopram,[22] which are being considered during JP's admission.

Table 3
Case 2 panel-based testing results

Genotype Results	Phenotype	Relevant Medication(s)	Reference(s)
HLA-B*15:02	Non-carrier	Oxcarbazepine	24
HLA-A*31:01	Non-carrier	Oxcarbazepine	24
CYP2D6 *1/*4	IM	Risperidone	25
CYP2C19 *1/*17	RM	Escitalopram	26
CYP2C9 *1/*1	NM	None	
CYP2B6 *1/*6	IM	None	
SLC6A4 S/S	Low Activity	None	27,28
HTR2A−1438 G > A G/A	Intermediate Activity	None	29

Relevant medication(s) refers to which medications are relevant to the case. Information about genes and results not featured in the case discussion can be found on PharmGKB.
Abbreviations: IM, intermediate metabolizer; NM, normal metabolizer; RM, rapid metabolizer.

JP's results for *HLA-B*15:02* and *HLA-A*31:01* inform his provider that oxcarbazepine is not contraindicated. Very serious cutaneous adverse reactions (eg, Stevens-Johnson Syndrome and toxic epidermal necrosis) can occur after treatment with carbamazepine or oxcarbazepine in patients carrying human leukocyte antigen (HLA) alleles *HLA-B*15:02* and *HLA-A*31:01*, which have variable frequency based on ethnic and geographical ancestry. CPIC recommends avoiding carbamazepine and oxcarbazepine in patients carrying one or more copies of these alleles.[21]

The CPIC guideline for SSRIs currently includes recommendations for escitalopram, based on CYP2C19 metabolizer status (**Fig. 3**).[22] Based on JP's CYP2C19 rapid metabolizer phenotype, standard escitalopram dosing is recommended.

Risperidone is metabolized by CYP2D6 into an active metabolite (9-hydroxyrisperidone or paliperidone). To determine if JP's CYP2D6 intermediate metabolizer status explained his past adverse reactions, JP's provider might search PharmGKB's Clinical Guideline Annotations to discover that while there is no CPIC guideline for risperidone,

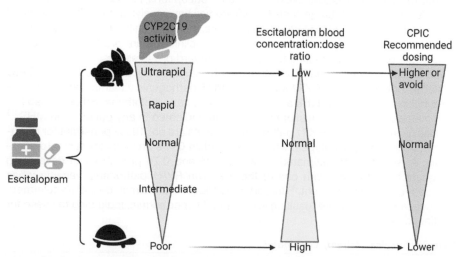

Fig. 3. Escitalopram dosing recommendations are based on CYP2C19 phenotype.[22] This figure was created using Biorender.com.

a Dutch Pharmacogenetics Working Group guideline recommends decreased dosing for CYP2D6 poor metabolizers. For CYP2D6 ultrarapid metabolizers, an alternative drug or titrating risperidone to the maximum dose for the active metabolite (paliperidone) is recommended.[23] Although dosing recommendations do not exist for CYP2D6 intermediate metabolizers, slower risperidone clearance may have contributed to JP's previous side effects.

Case 3a: Surgical Patient

CW is a 14-year-old male scheduled for vertebral body tethering for progressive scoliosis. CW previously participated in a research study during which genomic screening by a Clinical Laboratory Improvement Amendment (CLIA) certified and College of American Pathologists (CAP) accredited laboratory found a pathogenic variant in RYR1. The finding was disclosed to the adolescent and his mother, and the PDF report was placed in CW's electronic health record. During the preoperative clinic visit, CW's mother shared the report with the anesthesiologist. There was no known family history of exposure to anesthesia. CW previously tolerated pressure equalizer tube placement at 18 months and tonsillectomy at 3 years of age. What precautions are indicated by the finding of a pathogenic variant in RYR1?

A pathogenic variant (previously referred to as mutation) in the *RYR1* gene identifies CW as having malignant hyperthermia susceptibility (MHS), an autosomal dominant condition which may remain clinically silent until adequate exposure to a triggering drug agent. Pathogenic variants in the *CACNA1S* gene have been reported in ~1% of patients with malignant hyperthermia.[24] Exposure to volatile anesthetics or depolarizing neuromuscular blockers, particularly succinylcholine, or the combination of succinylcholine and a volatile anesthetic, can trigger life-threatening malignant hyperthermia.[25] Children can present differently than adults, delaying diagnosis.[26–28] Clinical testing of *RYR1* and *CACNA1S* for MHS is available but not routinely performed in clinical settings prior to surgeries.[29]

ES and GS are increasingly used for clinical diagnosis. The American College of Medical Genetics and Genomics (ACMG) recommends that regardless of indication for clinical ES/GS, analysis should routinely include specified genes known to inform genetic disorders with preventive or early treatment options, including *RYR1* and *CACNA1S* (since 2013).[30,31] Large scale ES/GS studies have analyzed the ACMG specified genes and provided results to study participants, including children.[32–34] As the use of clinical and research ES/GS increases, pediatric clinicians are prudent to add questions about prior genetic testing for MHS to standard pre-anesthesia assessments.

In our case, CW previously tolerated anesthesia. Even in cases like this, the CPIC guideline that includes 48 *RYR1* and 2 *CACNA1S* pathogenic variants states that succinylcholine and potent volatile anesthetics (sevoflurane, halothane, enflurane, isoflurane, methoxyflurane, and desflurane) are contraindicated in any patient with MHS.[35] Studies have shown that *RYR1* pathogenic variants are not 100% penetrant for malignant hyperthermia phenotypes, which may explain CW's previous tolerance to anesthesia. A recent study estimated between 0.25 and 0.76 probability of developing malignant hyperthermia with one of the 9 known *RYR1* pathogenic variants when exposed to a triggering agent.[36] Importantly, trigger agents may be initially tolerated, with subsequent exposure resulting in malignant hyperthermia, indicating the need for continued vigilance.[35]

Case 3b: Surgical Patient, Continued

CW's mother reported that after his prior tonsillectomy, oral codeine was ineffective. Of note, a prior hospitalization for major depression led to PGx panel testing, and he was found to be a CYP2D6 poor metabolizer (diplotype *3/*4) and CYP2C19 normal metabolizer (diplotype *1/*1). Current medications include sertraline daily for depression and cetirizine daily as needed for seasonal allergies. The orthopedic surgeon reviewed the psychiatry PGx report, noted recommendations for antidepressants and antipsychotics, and was uncertain about the implications for postoperative pain management. *How do these PGx results inform postoperative management?*

Opioids and nonsteroidal anti-inflammatory drugs (NSAIDs) are essential components of perioperative pain management.[37] Ondansetron is commonly prescribed as opioids increase postoperative nausea and vomiting. Variable CYP2D6 function can impact effectiveness and risk for adverse reactions for some opioids and may impact ondansetron efficacy. In our case, CW has *CYP2D6* *3/*4 genotype, with 2 no function alleles, consistent with a poor metabolizer phenotype. CW's results for CYP2D6 and CYP2C19 do not inform the use of NSAIDs, which are metabolized by CYP2C9 and discussed further in Case 4.

Codeine and tramadol are prodrugs (inactive in their dosage forms) and are O-demethylated by CYP2D6 to their active (analgesic) metabolites, morphine, and O-desmethyltramadol, respectively. CYP2D6 poor metabolizers cannot convert codeine or tramadol to their active forms, and codeine and tramadol will not provide pain relief. Evidence-based guidelines recommend avoiding codeine and tramadol in any CYP2D6 poor metabolizer (see **Fig. 1**A). If an opioid is required for pain management, then a non-tramadol and a non-codeine containing analgesic should be considered.[38]

The FDA issued a contraindication for codeine products and tramadol in all children less than 12 years of age, children less than 18 years after tonsillectomy or who are obese, have obstructive sleep apnea or lung disease.[39] Since then, the use of codeine has decreased and the use of oxycodone has increased in children.[2] Oxycodone and hydrocodone are converted by CYP2D6 to their more active metabolites, oxymorphone and hydromorphone. Although lower active drug concentrations are observed in CYP2D6 poor metabolizers, a clear clinical difference in drug response has not been demonstrated. Because past studies had few participants identified as CYP2D6 ultrarapid metabolizers, there is insufficient evidence regarding the safety and efficacy of oxycodone and hydrocodone for these individuals.[38] For CW, if opioids are required for post-operative pain management, standard dosing of oxycodone or hydrocodone would be appropriate.

Ondansetron, a 5-HT receptor antagonist, is used to prevent nausea and vomiting and is inactivated by CYP2D6. Evidence from clinical studies in adults indicates an alternative medication may be needed for CYP2D6 ultrarapid metabolizers due to inadequate effectiveness.[40] Standard dosing was effective and well tolerated by adult patients who were CYP2D6 intermediate or poor metabolizers. Studies in children at risk for postoperative nausea and vomiting are needed.[41,42] Further discussion of ondansetron is included in case 4 later in discussion.

Case 4: Oncology Patient

AR is a 16-year-old female diagnosed with acute lymphoblastic leukemia. Her tumor genetic testing indicated she had the BCR-ABL translocation, which means a tyrosine kinase inhibitor (eg, dasatinib or imatinib) is indicated. Her treatment regimen will also include mercaptopurine, ondansetron, opioids, and NSAIDs. She may receive voriconazole, tacrolimus, proton pump inhibitors (PPIs), and/or an SSRI. For these reasons, the oncology pharmacist orders a multi-gene PGx panel. A buccal swab was performed for her PGx panel, as a blood sample at the start of treatment would be largely leukemic cells that may have more mutations than her germline. The panel test results are shown in **Table 4**. The medications relevant to each gene on the medications she will receive are detailed later in discussion. *How might these PGx results inform her chemotherapy and symptomatic management?*

Thiopurines (eg, mercaptopurine) are inactive prodrugs that are metabolized into active immunosuppressants, which are then inactivated by the TPMT and NUDT15 enzymes. The CPIC guideline aligns with the FDA package insert for mercaptopurine, which indicates that TPMT or NUDT15 intermediate metabolizers often tolerate recommended standard mercaptopurine doses, but some require dose reduction based on toxicities.[43] If AR had been found to be a TPMT or NUDT15 poor metabolizer, her dose would need to be reduced dramatically (~10-fold). As most patients with leukemia in the U.S. are enrolled in clinical trials, the recommended dose of mercaptopurine based on TPMT and NUDT15 will be dictated by the study protocol.

Ondansetron and opioids were addressed in the previous case. However, in this case, AR is a CYP2D6 ultrarapid metabolizer. Ondansetron is prescribed to prevent or reduce chemotherapy-induced nausea and vomiting. As a CYP2D6 ultrarapid metabolizer, she metabolizes ondansetron quickly, and CPIC recommends an alternative antiemetic not metabolized by CYP2D6 (eg, granisetron),[40] though this is based on adult studies, and 2 recent studies in children could not replicate differences in response.[41,42] If opioids are needed for pain control, codeine and tramadol should be avoided because CYP2D6 ultrarapid metabolizers produce more of the active metabolite than normal metabolizers (see **Fig. 1**A), which puts them at increased risk of respiratory depression and other adverse events.[38] If pain can be controlled by NSAIDs, the patient's CYP2C9 result is relevant for some options (see **Table 4**). The patient is a normal metabolizer for CYP2C9, so she should receive the typical doses of these medications (**Fig. 4**).

The antifungal agent voriconazole may be used prophylactically or to treat a fungal infection. As this patient is a CYP2C19 intermediate metabolizer, CPIC recommends the usual starting dose with adjustments being made for clinical factors, such as drug interactions, hepatic function, renal function, fungal species, site of infection, therapeutic drug monitoring, and comorbidities (**Fig. 5**).[20] The patient will likely have higher dose-adjusted concentrations than normal metabolizers so may need a decreased dose after therapeutic drug monitoring.

Table 4
Case 4 Panel-based testing results

Genotype Results	Phenotype	Relevant Medication(s)	Reference(s)
CYP2D6 *1/*1x2	UM	Ondansetron, codeine, tramadol, paroxetine, fluvoxamine	9,31,48
CYP2C19 *1/*2	IM	Voriconazole, omeprazole, lansoprazole, pantoprazole, dexlansoprazole, sertraline, escitalopram, citalopram	10,31,51
CYP2C9 *1/*1	NM	Celecoxib, flurbiprofen, ibuprofen and lornoxicam	30
CYP3A5 *1/*3	IM	Tacrolimus	52
TPMT *1/*1	NM	Mercaptopurine	53
NUDT15 *1/*3	IM	Mercaptopurine	53

Relevant medication(s) refers to which medications are relevant to the case. Information about genes and results not featured in the case discussion can be found on PharmGKB.

Abbreviations: IM, intermediate metabolizer; NM, normal metabolizer; UM, ultrarapid metabolizer.

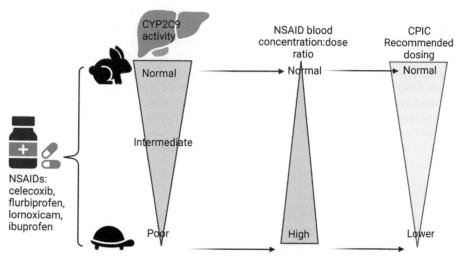

Fig. 4. Nonsteroidal anti-inflammatory drugs (NSAIDs) dosing recommendations are based on CYP2C9 phenotype.[20] Of note, CYP2C9 does not have any variants that would make a patient a rapid or ultrarapid metabolizer. This figure was created using Biorender.com.

PPIs (eg, omeprazole) may be prescribed to this patient prophylactically or for gastroesophageal reflux. As a CYP2C19 intermediate metabolizer, she should receive the usual dose at the start of therapy but consider a 50% reduced dose for chronic therapy more than 12 weeks due to increased risk for adverse events, including respiratory and gastrointestinal infections.[44] CYP2C19 rapid and ultrarapid metabolizers are likely to have reduced blood concentrations and could need higher doses (see **Fig. 1B**).

Tacrolimus may be considered for AR if she requires a hematopoietic stem cell transplant. *CYP3A5* variation explains ~50% of the variability in tacrolimus plasma

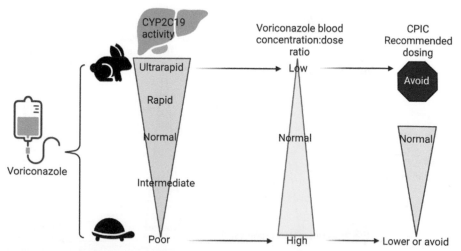

Fig. 5. Voriconazole recommendations are based on CYP2C19 phenotype.[59] This figure was created using Biorender.com.

concentrations.[45] Individuals who carry at least one *1 normal function allele (intermediate and normal metabolizers) are called expressers and those without are called non-expressers or poor metabolizers. The most common phenotype among individuals of European ancestry is poor metabolizer, and this epidemiology is what the usual dosing regimens are based on in the U.S. For expressers, CPIC recommends starting doses 1.5-2x higher than normal (though not exceeding 0.3 mg/kg/d), which should be followed by routine therapeutic drug monitoring (**Fig. 6**).[45] AR is an intermediate metabolizer so she would need a higher than normal starting dose of tacrolimus to prevent or treat graft-versus-host disease.

SSRIs are often prescribed to adolescent patients with cancer for depression and anxiety, and were previously discussed in Case 2.

Case 5: Patient with Rare Genetic Disease

ML is a 6-week-old infant who had a positive newborn screen for cystic fibrosis. After additional CFTR testing F508del/G542X and a confirmatory sweat test, ML is being evaluated by providers at an accredited CF center. ML's parents feel overwhelmed by the lifelong care ML will require but feel hopeful when they learn that ML's genetic results indicate ML will qualify for a new type of medication called CFTR modulators.

CFTR testing is recommended as part of the diagnostic process for cystic fibrosis (CF).[46] Pathogenic variants in the *CFTR* gene result in dysfunction or absence of the chloride ion channel, cystic fibrosis transmembrane conductance regulator. People with CF have pathogenic variants in each of their *CFTR* genes resulting in multiorgan disease manifestations.[47] Disease management had relied on symptom-based treatments with incremental improvement over the years in lifespan and quality of life.[48] *CFTR* testing has become an essential first step before prescribing a new class of drugs called CFTR modulators, considered transformational therapies as they address the molecular cause of CF. CFTR modulators are small molecules designed to restore or improve the function of certain types of variant CFTR protein.[47] There are over a 1000 pathogenic and likely pathogenic *CFTR* variants listed in ClinVar,[49] and each codes for one of the 6 classes of variant CFTR proteins.[50] Available

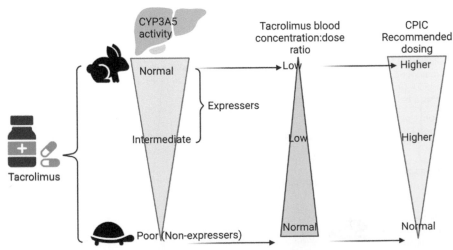

Fig. 6. Tacrolimus recommendations are based on CYP3A5 phenotype.[45] This figure was created using Biorender.com.

modulators target Class II, protein processing, and Class III gating variant CFTR.[47] The first FDA approved modulator, ivacaftor, is a potentiator. It helps the gating variant CFTR channel open at the cell membrane. Originally, it was approved for one specific pathogenic variant, G551D, found in less than 5% of patients with CF. Since then, its use has been expanded to include other gating variants in CFTR.[51]

ML has the most common pathogenic variant found in people with CF, F508del, and ML's other variant results in absent CFTR protein. Three FDA-approved modulators contain at least one corrector small molecule essential for patients who have F508del. CFTR correctors augment the protein folding process and transit to the cell membrane.[52] The most recently FDA-approved triple therapy modulator, elexa-caftor/tezacaftor/ivacaftor, has 2 CFTR correctors to maximize stable folding and transport of the F508del CFTR protein to the cell membrane and it has the potentiator to improve the gating function of the F508del protein. It is approved in children 6 years and older,[53] is considered lifelong, and costs over $300,000 per year in the U.S.[54] Health Canada Guidelines indicate elexacaftor/tezacaftor/ivacaftor will be the primary modulator therapy for any CF patient over the age of 12 who has at least one F508del variant.[55]

Throughout ML's life, multiple medications and therapies will be needed[48] to manage symptoms that may include PPIs (discussed above) and aminoglycosides for which CPIC guidelines are available. Specific variants in the mitochondrial gene, *MT-RNR1*, predispose individuals to severe aminoglycoside-induced hearing loss. A point-of-care *MT-RNR1* genotyping test has recently been developed for clinical use,[56] but testing is not done routinely due to the complexity of genotyping mitochondrial DNA. It is recommended that aminoglycoside antibiotics be avoided in individuals with one of the high-risk *MT-RNR1* variants unless the infection severity or lack of effective alternative therapies outweighs the risk of hearing loss.[57] Mitochondrial genes are maternally inherited. Because each cell in the body has hundreds to thousands of mitochondria and each mitochondrion has many copies of mitochondrial DNA,[58] genetic counseling should precede genetic testing.

CLINICS CARE POINTS

- Evidence-based gene-drug guidelines are freely available online through PharmGKB and CPIC; however, evidence specifically for children may be limited or absent.

- Potential for phenoconversion due to concomitant administration of inducers and inhibitors may need to be considered when using PGx test results to select or dose medications.
  - FDA Drug Development and Drug Interactions Table of Substrates, Inhibitors, and Inducers is a helpful resource

- Some pediatric health care facilities have or are building PGx clinical decision support into their EHRs, and these may or may not incorporate individualized phenoconversion adjustments to therapeutic recommendations.

- Some pediatric health care facilities have pharmacogenomic consultation services that may be managed by a pharmacy or a pharmacogenomic-specific multidisciplinary team.
  - Pediatric prescribers should find out what is available at their facility or local children's hospital.

- Pediatric providers should consider the following if they work at a facility that does not offer point-of-care clinical decision support or consultation services:
  - Identify commonly prescribed medications and proactively identify which of those medications have evidence-based guidelines and have the potential to be impacted by phenoconversion.

> o Identify a local or regional genetic counselor who might be able to help identify reputable laboratories offering PGx testing or who may be willing to schedule clinical encounters with patients interested in PGx testing. The National Society of Genetic Counselors is a good place to start (see **Table 2**).

DISCLOSURE

L.B. Ramsey serves as a consultant and has received grant funding from BTG Specialty Pharmaceuticals. L.B. Ramsey receives funding from the National Institutes of Health, United States (R01HD099775 and R01HD089928). C.A. Prows receives funding from the National Institutes of Health (U01 HG011172, R01HG010166) and is an inventor on Patent US 10,662,476 B2 - Personalized pain management and anesthesia: preemptive risk identification and therapeutic decision support but has not received any associated royalties. SLV receives funding from the National Institutes of Health (R01GM132204, U01HG010232, P50 HD106446). S.T. Girdwood receives funding from the National Institute of General Medical Sciences, United States (1R35GM146701).

REFERENCES

1. Relling MV, Klein TE, Gammal RS, et al. The Clinical Pharmacogenetics Implementation Consortium: 10 Years Later. Clin Pharmacol Ther 2020;107(1):171–5.
2. Ramsey LB, Ong HH, Schildcrout JS, et al. Prescribing Prevalence of Medications With Potential Genotype-Guided Dosing in Pediatric Patients. JAMA Netw Open 2020;3(12):e2029411.
3. Avello K, Bell M, Stein Q, et al. Perspectives of Pediatric Providers Regarding Clinical Use of Pharmacogenetics. S D Med 2021;74(7):294–301. Available at: https://pubmed.ncbi.nlm.nih.gov/34449988/. Accessed October 14, 2022.
4. Ramsey LB, Prows CA, Zhang K, et al. Implementation of Pharmacogenetics at Cincinnati Children's Hospital Medical Center: Lessons Learned Over 14 Years of Personalizing Medicine. Clin Pharmacol Ther 2019;105(1):49–52.
5. Brown JT, Ramsey LB, Van Driest SL, et al. Characterizing Pharmacogenetic Testing Among Children's Hospitals. Clin Transl Sci 2021;14(2):692–701.
6. Gregornik D, Salyakina D, Brown M, et al. Pediatric pharmacogenomics: challenges and opportunities: on behalf of the Sanford Children's Genomic Medicine Consortium. Pharmacogenomics J 2021;21(1):8–19.
7. Miller DT, Lee K, Gordon AS, et al. Recommendations for reporting of secondary findings in clinical exome and genome sequencing, 2021 update: a policy statement of the American College of Medical Genetics and Genomics (ACMG). Genet Med 2021;23(8):1391–8.
8. Ramsey LB, Brown JT, Vear SI, et al. Gene-based dose optimization in children. Annu Rev Pharmacol Toxicol 2020;60:311–31.
9. Gaedigk A, Ingelman-Sundberg M, Miller NA, et al. The Pharmacogene Variation (PharmVar) Consortium: Incorporation of the Human Cytochrome P450 (CYP) Allele Nomenclature Database. Clin Pharmacol Ther 2018;103(3):399–401.
10. Caudle KE, Dunnenberger HM, Freimuth RR, et al. Standardizing terms for clinical pharmacogenetic test results: Consensus terms from the Clinical Pharmacogenetics Implementation Consortium (CPIC). Genet Med 2017;19(2):215–23.
11. Caudle KE, Sangkuhl K, Whirl-Carrillo M, et al. Standardizing CYP2D6 Genotype to Phenotype Translation: Consensus Recommendations from the Clinical

Pharmacogenetics Implementation Consortium and Dutch Pharmacogenetics Working Group. Clin Transl Sci 2020;13(1):116–24.

12. Tang Girdwood SC, Rossow KM, Van Driest SL, et al. Perspectives from the Society for Pediatric Research: pharmacogenetics for pediatricians. Pediatr Res 2022;91(3):529–38.

13. Nicholson WT, Formea CM, Matey ET, et al. Considerations When Applying Pharmacogenomics to Your Practice. Mayo Clin Proc 2021;96(1):218–30.

14. Bousman CA, Zierhut H, Müller DJ. Navigating the Labyrinth of Pharmacogenetic Testing: A Guide to Test Selection. Clin Pharmacol Ther 2019;106(2):309–12.

15. Cicali EJ, Elchynski AL, Cook KJ, et al. How to Integrate CYP2D6 Phenoconversion Into Clinical Pharmacogenetics: A Tutorial. Clin Pharmacol Ther 2021;110(3):677–87.

16. Malki MA, Pearson ER. Drug-drug-gene interactions and adverse drug reactions. Pharmacogenomics J 2020;20(3):355–66.

17. Stout SM, Nemerovski CW, Streetman DS, et al. Interpretation of Cytochrome P-450 Inhibition and Induction Effects From Clinical Data: Current Standards and Recommendations for Implementation. Clin Pharmacol Ther 2021;109(1):82–6.

18. Hayashi M, Hamdy DA, Mahmoud SH. Applications for pharmacogenomics in pharmacy practice: A scoping review. Res Social Adm Pharm 2022;18(7):3094–118.

19. Gammal RS, Fieg E. Pharmacist and genetic counselor collaboration in pharmacogenomics. Am J Health Syst Pharm 2022;79(18). https://doi.org/10.1093/AJHP/ZXAC168.

20. Theken KN, Lee CR, Gong L, et al. Clinical Pharmacogenetics Implementation Consortium Guideline (CPIC) for CYP2C9 and Nonsteroidal Anti-Inflammatory Drugs. Clin Pharmacol Ther 2020;108(2):191–200.

21. Phillips EJ, Sukasem C, Whirl-Carrillo M, et al. Clinical Pharmacogenetics Implementation Consortium Guideline for HLA Genotype and Use of Carbamazepine and Oxcarbazepine: 2017 Update. Clin Pharmacol Ther 2018;103(4):574–81.

22. Bousman CA, Stevenson JM, Ramsey LB, et al. Clinical Pharmacogenetics Implementation Consortium (CPIC) Guideline for CYP2D6, CYP2C19, CYP2B6, SLC6A4, and HTR2A Genotypes and Serotonin Reuptake Inhibitor Antidepressants. Clin Pharmacol Ther 2023;114(1):51–68.

23. Risperidone. Available at: https://www.pharmgkb.org/chemical/PA451257/guidelineAnnotation/PA166104943. Accessed October 5, 2022.

24. Yang L, Dedkova EN, Allen PD, et al. T lymphocytes from malignant hyperthermia-susceptible mice display aberrations in intracellular calcium signaling and mitochondrial function. Cell Calcium 2021;93:102325.

25. Larach MG, Klumpner TT, Brandom BW, et al. Succinylcholine Use and Dantrolene Availability for Malignant Hyperthermia TreatmentDatabase Analyses and Systematic Review. Anesthesiology 2019;130(1):41–54.

26. Kim KSM, Kriss RS, Tautz TJ. Malignant Hyperthermia: A Clinical Review. Adv Anesth 2019;37:35–51.

27. Brandom BW, Bina S, Wong CA, et al. Ryanodine receptor type 1 gene variants in the malignant hyperthermia-susceptible population of the United States. Anesth Analg 2013;116(5):1078–86.

28. Nelson P, Litman RS. Malignant hyperthermia in children: An analysis of the north american malignant hyperthermia registry. Anesth Analg 2014;118(2):369–74.

29. Biesecker LG, Dirksen RT, Girard T, et al. Genomic Screening for Malignant Hyperthermia Susceptibility. Anesthesiology 2020;133(6):1277–82.

30. Miller DT, Lee K, Abul-Husn NS, et al. ACMG SF v3.1 list for reporting of secondary findings in clinical exome and genome sequencing: A policy statement of the American College of Medical Genetics and Genomics (ACMG). Genet Med 2022; 24(7):1407–14.

31. Green RC, Berg JS, Grody WW, et al. ACMG recommendations for reporting of incidental findings in clinical exome and genome sequencing. Genet Med 2013;15(7):565–74.

32. Ceyhan-Birsoy O, Ceyhan-Birsoy O, Murry JB, et al. Interpretation of Genomic Sequencing Results in Healthy and Ill Newborns: Results from the BabySeq Project. Am J Hum Genet 2019;104(1):76–93.

33. Myers MF, Martin LJ, Prows CA. Adolescents' and Parents' Genomic Testing Decisions: Associations With Age, Race, and Sex. J Adolesc Heal 2020;66(3): 288–95.

34. Hart MR, Biesecker BB, Blout CL, et al. Secondary findings from clinical genomic sequencing: prevalence, patient perspectives, family history assessment, and health-care costs from a multisite study. Genet Med 2019;21(5):1100–10.

35. Gonsalves SG, Dirksen RT, Sangkuhl K, et al. Clinical Pharmacogenetics Implementation Consortium (CPIC) Guideline for the Use of Potent Volatile Anesthetic Agents and Succinylcholine in the Context of RYR1 or CACNA1S Genotypes. Clin Pharmacol Ther 2019;105(6):1338–44.

36. Ibarra Moreno CA, Hu S, Kraeva N, et al. An Assessment of Penetrance and Clinical Expression of Malignant Hyperthermia in Individuals Carrying Diagnostic Ryanodine Receptor 1 Gene Mutations. Anesthesiology 2019;131(5):983–91.

37. Cravero JP, Agarwal R, Berde C, et al. The Society for Pediatric Anesthesia recommendations for the use of opioids in children during the perioperative period. Paediatr Anaesth 2019;29(6):547–71.

38. Crews KR, Monte AA, Huddart R, et al. Clinical Pharmacogenetics Implementation Consortium Guideline for CYP2D6, OPRM1, and COMT Genotypes and Select Opioid Therapy. Clin Pharmacol Ther 2021;110(4):888–96.

39. FDA (Food and Drug Administration). Safety Review Update of Codeine Use in Children; New Boxed Warning and Contraindication on Use after Tonsillectomy and/or Adenoidectomy. Available at: https://www.fda.gov/media/85072/download. Accessed March 31, 2020.

40. Bell GC, Caudle KE, Whirl-Carrillo M, et al. Clinical Pharmacogenetics Implementation Consortium (CPIC) guideline for CYP2D6 genotype and use of ondansetron and tropisetron. Clin Pharmacol Ther 2017;102(2). https://doi.org/10.1002/cpt.598.

41. Edwards A, Teusink-Cross A, Martin LJ, et al. Influence of CYP2D6 metabolizer status on ondansetron efficacy in pediatric patients undergoing hematopoietic stem cell transplantation: A case series. Clin Transl Sci 2022;15(3):610–8.

42. Black K, Brenn B, Gaedigk A, et al. Pediatric CYP2D6 Metabolizer Status and Post-Tonsillectomy Nausea and Vomiting After Ondansetron. Clin Transl Sci 2023;16(2):269–78.

43. Relling MV, Schwab M, Whirl-Carrillo M, et al. Clinical Pharmacogenetics Implementation Consortium Guideline for Thiopurine Dosing Based on TPMT and NUDT15 Genotypes: 2018 Update. Clin Pharmacol Ther 2019;105(5):1095–105.

44. Lima JJ, Thomas CD, Barbarino J, et al. Clinical Pharmacogenetics Implementation Consortium (CPIC) Guideline for CYP2C19 and Proton Pump Inhibitor Dosing. Clin Pharmacol Ther 2021;109(6):1417–23.

45. Birdwell KA, Decker B, Barbarino JM, et al. Clinical Pharmacogenetics Implementation Consortium (CPIC) guidelines for CYP3A5 genotype and tacrolimus dosing. Clin Pharmacol Ther 2015;98(1):19–24.

46. Farrell PM, White TB, Ren CL, et al. Diagnosis of Cystic Fibrosis: Consensus Guidelines from the Cystic Fibrosis Foundation. J Pediatr 2017;181:S4–15.e1.

47. Clancy JP, Cotton CU, Donaldson SH, et al. CFTR modulator theratyping: Current status, gaps and future directions. J Cyst Fibros 2019;18(1):22–34.

48. Borowitz D, Robinson KA, Rosenfeld M, et al. Cystic Fibrosis Foundation Evidence-Based Guidelines for Management of Infants with Cystic Fibrosis. J Pediatr 2009;155(6):S73–93.

49. ClinVar. Available at: https://www.ncbi.nlm.nih.gov/clinvar/. Accessed October 5, 2022.

50. Bareil C, Bergougnoux A. CFTR gene variants, epidemiology and molecular pathology. Arch Pediatr 2020;27(Suppl 1):eS8–12. https://doi.org/10.1016/S0929-693X(20)30044-0.

51. CPIC® Guideline for Ivacaftor and CFTR – CPIC. Available at: https://cpicpgx.org/guidelines/guideline-for-ivacaftor-and-cftr/. Accessed October 5, 2022.

52. Van Goor F, Hadida S, Grootenhuis PDJ, et al. Correction of the F508del-CFTR protein processing defect in vitro by the investigational drug VX-809. Proc Natl Acad Sci U S A 2011;108(46):18843–8.

53. fda, cder. TRIKAFTA HIGHLIGHTS OF PRESCRIBING INFORMATION. Available at: www.fda.gov/medwatch. Accessed October 5, 2022.

54. Guo J, Garratt A, Hill A. Worldwide rates of diagnosis and effective treatment for cystic fibrosis. J Cyst Fibros 2022;21(3):456–62.

55. Chilvers MA, Waters V, Anderson MR, et al. CANADIAN CLINICAL CONSENSUS GUIDELINE FOR INITIATION, MONITORING AND DISCONTINUATION OF CFTR MODULATOR THERAPIES FOR PATIENTS WITH CYSTIC FIBROSIS. Available at: https://hpr-rps.hres.ca/details.php?drugproductid=4285&query=kalydeco. Accessed October 5, 2022.

56. McDermott JH, Mahaveer A, James RA, et al. Rapid Point-of-Care Genotyping to Avoid Aminoglycoside-Induced Ototoxicity in Neonatal Intensive Care. JAMA Pediatr 2022;176(5):486–92.

57. McDermott JH, Wolf J, Hoshitsuki K, et al. Clinical Pharmacogenetics Implementation Consortium Guideline for the Use of Aminoglycosides Based on MT-RNR1 Genotype. Clin Pharmacol Ther 2022;111(2):366–72.

58. Craven L, Alston CL, Taylor RW, et al. Recent Advances in Mitochondrial Disease. Annu Rev Genomics Hum Genet 2017;18:257–75.

59. Moriyama B, Obeng AO, Barbarino J, et al. Clinical Pharmacogenetics Implementation Consortium (CPIC) Guidelines for CYP2C19 and Voriconazole Therapy. Clin Pharmacol Ther 2017;102(1):45–51.

Newborn Screening

Kara B. Pappas, MD[a,b],*

KEYWORDS

- Newborn screening • Inborn errors of metabolism • Hearing loss
- Congenital heart disease • Hemoglobinopathies • Immunodeficiency
- Galactosemia • Endocrine disorders

KEY POINTS

- Newborn screening is performed in order to identify health conditions in which early treatment can improve the outcome.
- Newborn screening in the United States consists of both tests on dried blood spots and point-of-care testing.
- Point-of-care testing screens for hearing loss and congenital heart disease.
- Screening is done on dried blood spots for various inborn errors of metabolism, hemoglobinopathies, endocrine disorders, immunodeficiencies, cystic fibrosis, and neurologic disorders.
- Pediatricians play a vital role in newborn screening and help ensure timely diagnosis, treatment, and referrals of patients for specialty care.

INTRODUCTION TO NEWBORN SCREENING

Newborn screening refers to a diverse set of tests that are done on newborns in order to identify disorders in which early treatment can improve the outcome. Point-of-care testing includes screening for hearing loss and screening for critical congenital heart disease. Dried blood spots are taken typically in the first few days of life, and many different tests are done to screen for various inborn errors of metabolism, endocrine disorders, cystic fibrosis, neurologic disorders, hemoglobinopathies, and immunologic disorders.

In the United States, there is a Recommended Uniform Screening Panel (RUSP) for disorders recommended by the Department of Health and Human Services (**Table 1**). The individual states and newborn screening centers have the flexibility to change this list, however most screen for at least the recommended disorders. States may use different methods and cut-offs for screening, leading to differences in diagnosis and

a Division of Genetics, Genomics and Metabolic Disorders, Children's Hospital of Michigan, Detroit, MI, USA; b Department of Pediatrics, Central Michigan University, Mount Pleasant, MI, USA
* Division of Genetics, Genomics and Metabolic Disorders, Children's Hospital of Michigan, 3950 Beaubien Street, 4th floor, Detroit, MI 48201.
E-mail address: Kpappas@dmc.org

Pediatr Clin N Am 70 (2023) 1013–1027
https://doi.org/10.1016/j.pcl.2023.06.003
0031-3955/23/© 2023 Elsevier Inc. All rights reserved.

pediatric.theclinics.com

Table 1
Recommended uniform screening panel

Category	Core Conditions	Secondary Conditions
Metabolic: Organic Acid Disorder	Propionic Acidemia Methylmalonic Acidemia (mutase) Methylmalonic Acidemia (cobalamin disorders) Isovaleric Acidemia 3-Methylcrotonyl-CoA Carboxylase Deficiency 3-Hydroxy-3-Methylglutaric Aciduria Holocarboxylase Synthase Deficiency Beta-ketothiolase Deficiency Glutaric Acidemia Type I	Methylmalonic acidemia with homocystinuria Malonic acidemia Isobutyrylglycinuria 2-Methylbutyrylglycinuria 3-Methylglutaconic aciduria 2-Methyl-3-hydroxybutyric aciduria
Metabolic: Fatty Acid Oxidation Disorder	Carnitine Uptake Defect Medium-chain Acyl-CoA Dehydrogenase Deficiency Very Long-chain Acyl-CoA Dehydrogenase Deficiency Long-chain L-3 Hydroxyacyl-CoA Dehydrogenase Deficiency Trifunctional Protein Deficiency	Short-chain acyl-CoA dehydrogenase deficiency Medium/short-chain L-3-hydroxyacyl-CoA dehydrogenase deficiency Glutaric acidemia type II Medium-chain ketoacyl-CoA thiolase deficiency 2,4 Dienoyl-CoA reducatse deficiency Carnitine palmitoyltransferase type 1 deficiency Carnitine palmitoyltransferase type 2 deficiency Carnitine acylcarnitine translocase deficiency
Metabolic: Amino Acid Disorder	Arginosuccinic Aciduria Citrullinemia Type 1 Maple Syrup Urine Disease Homocytinuria Classic Phenylketonuria Tyrosinemia Type 1	Argininemia Citrullinemia Type 2 Hypermethioninemia Benign hyperphenylalaninemia Biopterin defect in cofactor synthesis Biopterin defect in cofactor regeneration Tyrosinemia type 2 Tyrosinemia type 3

Endocrine disorder	Primary Congenital Hypothyroidism
	Congenital Adrenal Hyperplasia
Hemoglobin Disorder	S,S Disease (Sickle Cell Anemia)	Other hemoglobinopathies
	S, C Disease
	S, Beta-Thalassemia
Other	Classic Galactosemia	Galactoepimerase deficiency
	Biotinidase Deficiency	Galactokinase deficiency
	Severe Combined Immunodeficiency	T-cell-related lymphocyte deficiencies
	Cystic Fibrosis
	Mucopolysaccharidosis Type I
	Mucopolysaccharidosis Type II
	Glycogen Storage Disease Type II (Pompe)
	X-linked Adrenoleukodystrophy
	Spinal Muscular Atrophy (due to exon 7 deletion)
	Hearing Loss
	Critical Congenital Heart Disease

ultimately treatment. It must be remembered that newborn screening is a screen and not a diagnosis; therefore confirmatory testing must take place after a positive screen is received.

This article will briefly describe the various disorders or groups of disorders tested, including methods and clinical considerations for pediatricians.

DISORDERS ON THE NEWBORN SCREEN

In this section, we will review the various types of disorders that are on the newborn screen. We will briefly describe the disease pathophysiology, clinical manifestations, treatment, screening methods, and confirmatory testing.

Hearing loss

Neonatal hearing loss has a variety of both genetic and environmental etiologies. Genetic etiologies may be syndromic (involving other birth defects or health concerns) or non-syndromic (isolated hearing loss). Common environmental causes include congenital infections (ie CMV), prematurity, medication exposure, and more. Diagnosis and treatment of early hearing loss is imperative for proper language development.

Newborn screening for hearing loss is recommended in the first few days of life, prior to hospital discharge. Two methods can be used. The first is otoacoustic emissions (OAE). An OAE is performed by placing a small probe in the ear canal, which delivers a sound to the auditory system. A microphone on the probe picks up the response by the cochlea, if present. OAE screening can have false positives particularly if there is debris or fluid in the middle ear or external auditory canal, which can be common in early life. OAE testing will not pick up hearing dysfunction due to problems with the auditory nerve or the auditory cortex, which may be damaged by certain postnatal exposures.

The second screening method is the Auditory Brainstem Response (ABR). An ABR is performed by placing electrodes on the forehead, providing sound, and noting brain activity response. ABR can detect hearing impairment originating anywhere along the auditory tract.

Hospitals may use one or both tests for hearing screens; some may use OAEs in low-risk babies and ABRs in high-risk babies, or may perform an ABR if a baby fails their initial OAE. If a baby ultimately fails their hearing screen, they are referred for further testing, typically to an Audiologist for further testing.[1]

Critical congenital heart disease

Newborn screening for Critical Congenital Heart Disease (CCHD) involves measuring both pre-ductal and post-ductal oxygen saturations. CCHD is not all encompassing; the purpose is to identify cardiac defects in which early treatment can prevent death or other morbidities; see **Table 2**. Some congenital heart defects can be detected

Table 2 Critical congenital heart defects	
• Coarctation of the aorta	• Single ventricle
• Double outlet right ventricle	• Tetralogy of Fallot
• Ebstein anomaly	• Total anomalous pulmonary venous return
• Hypoplastic left heart syndrome	• Transposition of the great arteries
• Interrupted aortic arch	• Tricuspid artresia
• Pulmonary atresia	• Truncus ateriosus

prenatally (estimated around 2/3), however the postnatal exam will often miss any unknown defects.[2] It is preferred to screen the baby after 24 hours of life to decrease false positive results, however, it is acceptable to screen earlier if the baby is being discharged.

CCHD screening is performed by placing a pulse oximeter on the right hand (preductal) and either foot (post-ductal). In general, a baby "passes" if the oxygen saturation is greater than 95% in both sites, and there is less than a 3% difference between the sites. If these conditions are not met, the baby may be rescreened or failed, at which time further testing may be done. Most states use an algorithm endorsed by the American Academy of Pediatrics, although there have been some recent recommendations to simplify this algorithm to reduce misinterpretation and decrease time to treatment.[3]

Confirmatory testing may include a chest radiograph, electrocardiogram and/or an echocardiogram with Cardiology involvement. Treatment is individualized to each defect and may include surgical repair.

CCHD is rather non-invasive and easy to perform. Hypoxemia detected on CCHD may also identify other hypoxic conditions, such as sepsis or lung disease.[2]

Hemoglobinopathies

The hemoglobinopathies encompass a diverse group of disorders that broadly affect the alpha-globin and beta-globin genes, affecting the production of hemoglobin. Sickle cell disorders include those with the abnormal structure of hemoglobin, whereas thalassemias are due to diminished amounts of normal alpha- or beta-globin chains.[4] Sickle cell anemia, Hemoglobin SC disease, and Sickle cell thalassemia are primary targets for newborn screening in the US, however other disorders are also found.

Sickle cell disease is due to pathogenic variants that cause abnormal shape of hemoglobin. This causes chronic hemolysis and vaso-occlusion, which can occur all over the body including the spleen. Splenic infarction leads to higher risk of infection and sepsis. Many other complications can occur including acute chest syndrome, pain crises, retinopathy, avascular necrosis, strokes, and more. Treatment may include penicillin prophylaxis, additional vaccines, hydroxyurea (which induces Hemoglobin F, leading to longer lifespan of the hemoglobin), splenectomy, and careful screening and management of the other potentially serious complications. Bone marrow transplant is used in some severe cases, and gene therapy is emerging as a treatment.[5]

Thalassemias can cause varying degrees of severity of anemia. The most severe, beta thalassemia major, causes severe anemia, bone marrow expansion (leading to bony abnormalities), splenic enlargement, chronic hemolysis, and heart failure. Treatment is similar to SCD, in addition to often including regular blood transfusions.[6]

Sickle cell plus other abnormal hemoglobin shapes (such as in Hemoglobin C) or in combination with a thalassemia can cause many of the same concerns as above, which is why they are targets for newborn screening as well.

Newborn screening for hemoglobinopathies is typically done with high-performance liquid chromatography, followed by another method to verify the result. Confirmatory testing may include similar testing, as well as parental testing, electrophoresis, and molecular methods depending on which disease is suspected.[4] Of note many places offer prenatal screening for various hemoglobinopathies depending on risk from family history of ethnicity.

Endocrine disorders

There are currently two endocrine disorders included on newborn screening, congenital hypothyroidism, and congenital adrenal hyperplasia.

Congenital hypothyroidism

Congenital hypothyroidism can lead to multiple abnormalities but these can be subtle at first. Poor feeding, constipation, lethargy, and prolonged hyperbilirubinemia are some of the more common findings in neonates. Some babies may have physical manifestations such as macroglossia, umbilical hernias, and a widened posterior fontanel. Delay in treatment can lead to poor growth and irreversible neurologic damage.[7]

Congenital hypothyroidism may be screened for with either TSH or T4 as the primary analyte, or both. Depending on how the test is designed, certain types of hypothyroidism could be missed; for example, central hypothyroidism may be missed by a T4-only NBS. There are changes in both TSH and T4 levels early in life, so attention must be paid to age-related cut-offs. The main cause of congenital hypothyroidism is thyroid dysgenesis, including hypoplasia or aplasia of the thyroid gland, or ectopic thyroid glands. Disorders of hormone synthesis can occur (both of TSH and thyroid hormone), or rarer conditions which could involve the transport or metabolism of the involved hormones or receptors. There are also a variety of causes of transient hypothyroidism including iodine deficiency and maternal antibodies. Confirmatory labs are typically TSH and T4, and are performed between 1 and 2 weeks of life. Treatment goals for congenital hypothyroidism are to normalize the T4 within 2 weeks, and the TSH within 1 month.[8]

Congenital adrenal hyperplasia

Congenital adrenal hyperplasia (CAH) encompasses multiple disorders of cortisol synthesis. Newborn screening checks for the most common type, 21-hydroxylase deficiency. 21-hydroxylase has two roles, involved in both cortisol and aldosterone production. Classic CAH due to 21-hydroxylase deficiency can cause 1) androgen excess, which may manifest as ambiguous genitalia in females and 2) aldosterone deficiency, which may lead to salt wasting and subsequent hypovolemia and potentially shock. There are milder forms that can cause a spectrum of features.

Newborn screening for CAH is typically performed by measuring the level of 17-hydroxyprogesterone (17-OHP). 17-OHP can be falsely elevated in preterm babies and babies who are otherwise critically ill. Values for 17-OHP may be adjusted for multiple factors including birth weight or gestational age. Some states may use a second-tier test to confirm the elevated 17-OHP or a second newborn screen.[9] Confirmatory testing typically includes 17-OHP, other hormones, and molecular methods.

Immediate treatment is necessary to prevent complications from the severe or salt-wasting form of CAH. Treatment may include glucocorticoids, mineralocorticoids, and salt supplementation. Other treatment may include the management of the ambiguous genitalia. Milder forms may not require treatment unless signs or symptoms present.[8]

Immunologic disorders

Severe combined immunodeficiency (SCID) is a condition in which there is lack of T cells, with other immune cells potentially missing, depending on the underlying cause. It is one of the most severe immunodeficiencies and can cause severe infections and early death without treatment. There are a large number of genes that can cause a SCID phenotype.

Newborn screening for SCID involves screening for the level of T cell receptor excision circles (TRECs), which are small pieces of DNA formed during T cell rearrangements. Patients screen positive if they have low TREC levels. However, this can also identify other disorders that cause low T cells, such as other immunodeficiencies, other genetic disorders (such as 22q11.2 deletion syndrome), certain congenital anomalies, and maternal diseases. There are a few types of SCID which may not be identified based on TREC levels including those that cause defects in T cell function rather than numbers.[10]

Confirmatory testing may include a number of immunologic tests. Hematopoietic stem cell transplant performed early often provides the best outcome. Other treatments depending on the defect may include avoidance of infection, immunoglobulin replacement, antimicrobial prophylaxis, or other medications. Gene therapy is also being studied.[11]

Cystic fibrosis

Cystic fibrosis (CF) is a disorder that causes primarily pulmonary disease and pancreatic insufficiency. CF is caused by the dysfunction of the cystic fibrosis transmembrane conductance regulator (CFTR) gene, which is involved in the transport of chloride and sodium across cell membranes. If transport is defective, buildup of thick secretions occurs, leading to clinical manifestations. Decreased mucocilary clearance in the respiratory tract leads to chronic airway obstruction, recurrent infections, and inflammatory damage. In the GI tract, there is impaired flow of bile and pancreatic secretions which leads to pancreatic insufficiency, malabsorption, and liver dysfunction. Meconium ileus, failure to thrive, diabetes, biliary obstruction, gastrointestinal obstruction, rectal prolapse, and male infertility can occur as well.[12]

Newborn screening for cystic fibrosis in the United States starts with an increased immunoreactive trypsinogen (IRT) level, which is a protein made by the pancreas. Typically, the samples with the highest levels are sent for further testing. Many states proceed to molecular testing for common pathogenic variants in *CFTR*. Some request a repeat specimen between 1 and 2 weeks of life, with or without molecular testing. Note it is important that the molecular test adequately cover the common pathogenic variants seen in the population being tested, which may change based on ethnic background and/or race.[13]

Confirmatory testing on those who screen positive must then take place. A sweat chloride test is the gold standard for the diagnosis of CF. Further genetic testing may be done as well. Treatment may include methods to enhance airway clearance, aggressive treatment of respiratory infections, airway anti-inflammatory treatment, pancreatic enzyme replacement therapy, replacement of fat-soluble vitamins, optimizing nutrition, and more. There are also CFTR modulator medications in patients with specific variants in CFTR which help enhance the activity of CFTR.[12]

Inborn errors of metabolism

There was a large increase in the number of disorders on the newborn screen with the application of the technology tandem mass spectroscopy (MS/MS). MS/MS allows the detection of multiple analytes quickly and easily that are markers for a variety of disorders including organic acidemias, fatty acid oxidation disorders, urea cycle disorders, and amino acid disorders.[14] These disorders often cause problems due to build up of toxic metabolites (such as organic acids, or ammonia), deficiency of energy production (such as hypoglycemia seen in fatty acid oxidation disorders), or both. A brief review of each group of disorders follows.

Amino acid disorders
Amino Acid Disorders, as their name implies, are caused by a deficiency in the breakdown or metabolism of amino acids. Examples include phenylketonuria (PKU, due to defects in metabolizing phenylalanine) and tyrosinemia (due to defects in the breakdown of tyrosine). Amino acid disorders have varying presentations, but are often

insidious in onset. They may cause non-specific developmental delays and other neurologic issues, liver problems, other health problems, and can cause characteristic odors (rotten cabbage in the case of tyrosinemia type 1).

Amino acids disorders are screened for by measuring amino acid levels via MS/MS. Confirmatory testing may include re-measuring amino acid levels along with other metabolic testing and genetic testing. Treatment often includes the restriction of the offending amino acid in the diet, and supplemental metabolic formula. A variety of medications are used which may reduce toxic buildup of metabolites, or work as co-factors to improve enzyme activity.[15]

Organic acidemias

Organic Acidemias (OA) are conditions due to defects in amino acid metabolism, either due to deficient enzyme, cofactor, or transporters. Examples include methylmalonic acidemia and propionic acidemia. Due to the defect, organic acids are produced with can cause a variety of downstream effects on organ function and other metabolic pathways. Babies often present in the first week of life with poor feeding, vomiting, lethargy, and can progress to seizures, coma, and death. Labs will usually reveal an anion gap metabolic acidosis, often with ketosis, lactic acidosis, and/or hyperammonemia. Multi-organ dysfunction occurs and features can include chronic kidney disease, cardiomyopathy, liver disease, recurrent pancreatitis, epilepsy, developmental delays, cytopenias, and more.

Organic acid disorders are screened for by measuring acylcarnitine levels via MS/MS. Confirmatory testing may include the measurement of acylcarnitines, amino acids, organic acids (often in the urine), other cofactor levels, enzyme activity, and genetic testing. Treatment typically includes a protein-restricted diet, supplemental metabolic formula, and a variety of medications that help reduce the toxic metabolites. Emergency care is also important, and most patients will have an emergency care plan outlining sick day plans.[16]

Urea cycle disorders

Patients with urea cycle disorders will present with hyperammonemia, as the urea cycle's main job is to rid the body of nitrogenous waste. Those with more severe forms of urea cycle disorders will present shortly after birth with signs of hyperammonemia such as lethargy, poor feeding, and vomiting, as well as respiratory alkalosis. Cerebral edema may occur leading to come and respiratory failure. Patients with urea cycle disorders are at risk for hyperammonemia during times of illness or with the ingestion of too much protein.

There are several urea cycle disorders on the RUSP, also classified as amino acid disorders, as they are due to defects in amino acid metabolism through the urea cycle. These disorders can also cause liver dysfunction and chronic neurologic abnormalities. These disorders are screened for by measuring amino acid levels on MS/MS. Confirmatory testing may include amino acid levels, urine tests, enzyme levels, and/ or genetic testing. Immediate treatment of hyperammonemia is necessary for the best outcome. Treatment includes protein-restricted diet, supplemental metabolic formula, medications to reduce ammonia levels, and supplemental amino acids as needed.[17]

Fatty acid oxidation disorders

Fatty acid oxidation disorders (FAOD) result from a defect in one of the many steps in beta-oxidation (break down of fatty acids to energy), or due to a defect in shuttling fatty acids into the mitochondria (the carnitine system). Fatty acids are essential for energy production during times of fasting, or of significant stress such as illness.

The heart and skeletal muscle also depend heavily on fatty acid oxidation for energy. FAOD can lead to hypoglycemia during long fasts or illnesses, which can in turn lead to seizures, coma, and permanent neurologic damage. Some FAOD can also lead to liver dysfunction, cardiomyopathy, cardiac arrhythmias, rhabdomyolysis, neuropathy, and ophthalmologic problems.

FAOD are screened for on the NBS via the acylcarnitine profile by MS/MS. Elevations of certain acylcarnitine compounds indicate different fatty acid oxidation disorders. Confirmatory testing usually involves repeating the acylcarnitine profile, urine tests, and carnitine levels. Functional testing, enzymatic testing, and genetic testing may be sent as well.

Treatment of FAOD involves three main facets, which depend on the disorder. First is the restriction of fats in some disorders, with the provision of "safe" fats such as medium-chain triglycerides to provide additional energy. Second is the supplementation of carnitine if low, which is essential for the metabolism of long-chain fats. Third is avoidance of fasting for long periods of time. Patients with FAOD must also have careful emergency management.[18]

Biotinidase deficiency

Biotinidase deficiency is a disorder due to a defect in the recycling of protein-bound biotin. Biotin is a cofactor for four enzymes important in various pathways, particularly protein metabolism. Patients with severe forms of biotinidase deficiency can present with neurologic abnormalities such as seizures and hypotonia, metabolic acidosis, vision loss, hearing loss, rashes and alopecia.

Biotinidase deficiency is screened for on the newborn screen by measuring the Biotinidase enzyme. Confirmatory testing includes enzyme testing and molecular testing. Treatment is provision of biotin supplementation and if patients remain on treatment, outcome is excellent.[16]

Galactosemia

Galactosemia is a condition due to a defect in the ability to convert galactose to glucose via the enzyme galactose-1-phosphate uridyltransferase (GALT). Galactose is found in many foods but most commonly in dairy products as it is part of lactose. The result is the accumulation of toxic metabolites. Untreated infants may develop feeding and growth issues, liver dysfunction, jaundice, bleeding, cataracts, E coli sepsis, and neurologic issues.

Newborn screening for galactosemia is done either by measuring the enzymatic activity of the GALT enzyme, measuring total and/or free galactose, or a combination of these. Confirmatory testing typically includes the testing of the GALT enzyme, galactose-1-phosphate levels, and molecular testing.

Treatment for galactosemia is a lactose-restricted diet. After starting this diet, the severe complications will resolve. However, even patients started on dietary treatment at an early age can still develop health issues including developmental delays (particularly in speech), motor problems and premature ovarian failure. There are mild variants of galactosemia that may not require any treatment.[19]

Lysosomal storage disorders

Lysosomal storage disorders (LSD) are a heterogeneous group of conditions due to defects in the lysosome, which performs many functions including the breakdown of complex molecules. In lysosomal storage disorders, complex molecules build up and cause organ damage. Clinical features vary widely however neurologic problems, ophthalmologic problems, organomegaly, and musculoskeletal problems are common. There is treatment for some lysosomal storage disorders making them more amenable to newborn screening. Enzyme replacement therapy involves regular infusions of the deficient enzyme. Other medications that lower buildup of molecules, hematopoietic stem cell transplant, and gene therapies are other treatment options.

Currently, on the RUSP, there are three LSDs: Mucopolysaccharidosis type 1 (also known as Hurler syndrome), Mucopolysaccharidosis type 2 (also known as Hunter syndrome), and Pompe disease (also a glycogen storage disease). Various states have added a number of other LSDs including Krabbe disease, Fabry disease, and Gaucher disease.

Newborn screening for LSDs involves the testing of the actual enzymatic activity through various methods. For some disorders an additional analyte or second-tier test may be used, including molecular testing. Confirmatory testing typically includes enzyme activity, urine tests for storage molecules, and molecular testing.[20]

Adrenoleukodystrophy

X-linked adrenoleukodystrophy (X-ALD) is a progressive disorder that can affect the nervous system and adrenal glands. X-ALD is a disorder of peroxisomal metabolism, and increased levels of very long-chain fatty acids are seen. As this is an X-linked disorder, males are affected more severely and can present severe progressive neurologic disease. First signs are typically learning and behavior problems between ages 4 and 8 years of age, which can quickly progress to severe intellectual disability, vision and hearing loss, seizures, spasticity, and loss of ambulation. The brain MRI findings of leukodystrophy often appear prior to the first clinical symptoms. Hematopoietic stem cell transplantation early in the development of neurologic disease can greatly improve outcomes. Males found to have X-ALD must be carefully monitored with clinical exams and brain imaging in order to provide the therapy when indicated and promote the best outcome. Males can have other phenotypes including myelopathy and adrenal insufficiency. Females with X-ALD can have neurologic symptoms later in life consistent with a myelopathy.

Newborn screening for X-ALD involves the screening of one of the very long-chain fatty acid levels. Males who screen positive are typically referred for evaluation. Confirmatory testing typically includes the measurement of very long chain fatty acid levels and molecular testing. Multiple specialists are often involved including Neurology, Endocrinology, and Genetics.[21] Females are not at immediate risk, but may be referred for counseling and testing of at-risk male relatives.

Spinal muscular atrophy

Spinal Muscular Atrophy (SMA) is a progressive neuromuscular disease. SMA is caused by the dysfunction of the survival motor neuron 1 (*SMN1*) gene, which helps maintain motor neurons. Deletion of exon 7 in the *SMN1* gene is the major cause of disease. There are various types of SMA classified based on severity and age of onset, with type 0 and 1 being the most severe. Children with the severe types of SMA either don't achieve or quickly lose motor milestones, and typically die in the first few years of life.

Newborn screening for SMA is done by screening for the common exon 7 deletion.[22] This means that a small percentage of children with SMA due to other mechanisms will be missed. Confirmatory testing is done with molecular analysis. Referral for further workup by Neurology and Genetics is crucial to confirm the diagnosis and initiate treatment. Various treatments are now available including gene enhancing and gene replacement therapy, which have had success if started presymptomatically.[23]

PRACTICAL CONSIDERATIONS IN NEWBORN SCREENING
Newborn screening process

The dried blood spot card is typically collected between 24 and 48 hours of life. It is important that the card then get transported to the state laboratory in a timely manner, typically within 24 hours of collection, so that testing can begin. The goal is to have results by 5 days of life for critical disorders, and 7 days for the remaining disorders.[24]

Some states require a second newborn screen to be sent, usually at 1 to 2 weeks of life, as some disorders may be easier to identify after some time has passed.[14]

A positive newborn screen

Pediatricians are typically the first person contacted regarding a positive newborn screen. Therefore pediatricians often must disclose the potential diagnosis, and help guide the parents to obtain confirmatory testing. Most of the time, patients are referred to appropriate specialists to work up the potential conditions. For some conditions in which there can be serious morbidity and/or mortality quickly, patients may be referred directly to the hospital for admission, workup, and treatment. In some states, there may be a referral center that helps coordinate disclosure and coordination of care.

Although confirmatory testing is often directed by specialists, there are resources regarding the appropriate lab testing to order after a positive newborn screen. These are provided by the American College of Medical Genetics. An example is the algorithm for Pompe disease (**Fig. 1**). In addition, the newborn screening laboratory will provide information to the pediatrician regarding the positive screen, the disorder, and information on what to do next, which may include repeating the newborn screen or referring the patient for further workup.

It is important to remember that many times, parents are not well educated on the purpose of newborn screening prior to the newborn screen being performed. As newborn screening is done in the first few days of life, often parents are exhausted and overwhelmed. Depending on the staff and place of birth, little education regarding the newborn screen may be done. It can be even more difficult to understand because in most cases, the babies appear healthy and "normal," as the disorder has not yet manifested. It is with special care and compassion that disclosure of a positive newborn screen must be delivered to parents or caretakers.

Special circumstances in newborn screening

There are a number of factors that can affect a newborn screen, which providers should be aware of. Humidity and heat can affect certain assays, particularly enzyme assays (such as Biotinidase activity), and can falsely lower the result. If a particular newborn screening card takes longer to get to the newborn screening lab under these conditions, it is possible to have a false positive newborn screen. Specimens are lost from time-to-time, and mix-ups can occur. This is why it is always important to get confirmatory testing.

Normal values of newborn screening analytes also change over time. Analytes may drastically increase or decrease in the first few days of life, so if a baby is screened after the recommended 24 to 48 hours, different cut-offs may be referenced. Premature babies, particularly those who are very premature, may screen positive for disorders simply because the normal ranges are unknown in their age group.

In addition, other factors may influence newborn screening analytes including total parental nutrition (TPN) and certain medications. Many states repeat the newborn screen during the NICU stay, or when a baby is discharged from the NICU, which

Pompe disease: acid alpha-glucosidase deficiency

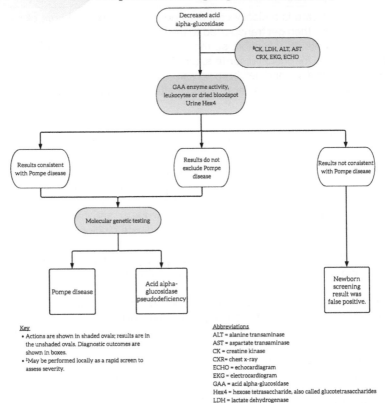

Key
- Actions are shown in shaded ovals; results are in the unshaded ovals. Diagnostic outcomes are shown in boxes.
- ‡May be performed locally as a rapid screen to assess severity.

Abbreviations
ALT = alanine transaminase
AST = aspartate transaminase
CK = creatine kinase
CXR = chest x-ray
ECHO = echocardiogram
EKG = electrocardiogram
GAA = acid alpha-glucosidase
Hex4 = hexose tetrasaccharide, also called glucotetrasaccharides
LDH = lactate dehydrogenase

Disclaimer: This practice resource is designed primarily as an educational resource for medical geneticists and other clinicians to help them provide quality medical services. Adherence to this practice resource is completely voluntary and does not necessarily assure a successful medical outcome. This practice resource should not be considered inclusive of all proper procedures and tests or exclusive of other procedures and tests that are reasonably directed to obtaining the same results. In determining the propriety of any specific procedure or test, the clinician should apply his or her own professional judgment to the specific clinical circumstances presented by the individual patient or specimen. Clinicians are encouraged to document the reasons for the use of a particular procedure or test, whether or not it is in conformance with this practice resource. Clinicians also are advised to take notice of the date this practice resource was adopted, and to consider other medical and scientific information that becomes available after that date. It also would be prudent to consider whether intellectual property interests may restrict the performance of certain tests and other procedures.

Fig. 1. Pompe disease: acid alpha-glucosidase deficiency. Key: • A ctions are show n in shaded ovals; results are in the unshaded ovals. Diagnostic outcomes are show n in boxes. • ?M ay be per for med locally as a rapid screen to assess sever ity. ALT, alanine transaminase; AST, aspar tate transaminase; CK, creatine kinase; CXR, chest x-ray; ECHO, echocar diagram; EKG, electrocar diogram; GA A, acid alpha-glucosidase; Hex4, hexose tetrasacchar ide, also called glucotetrasacchar ides; LDH, lactate dehydrogenase Disclaimer: This practice resource is designed primarily as an educational resource for medical geneticists and other clinicians to help them prov ide quality medical serv ices. A dherence to this practice resource is completely voluntary and does not necessarily assure a successful medical outcome. This practice resource should not be considered inclusive of all proper procedures and tests or exclusive of other procedures and tests that are reasonably directed to obtaining the same results. In determining the propriety of any specific procedure or test, the clinician should apply his or her ow n professional judgment to the specific clinical circumstances presented by the indiv idual patient or specimen. Clinicians are encouraged to document the reasons for the use of a particular procedure or test, w hether or not it is in conformance w ith this practice resource. Clinicians also are adv ised to take notice of the date this practice resource w as adopted, and to consider other medical and scientific information that becomes available after that date. It also w ould be prudent to consider w hether intellectual property interests may restrict the performance of certain tests and other procedures. © A mer ican College of M edical Genetics and Genomics, 2022 Cont ent Updat ed: July 2022 (Funded in part through M CHB/HRSA/HHS grant #U22 M C03957;#UH9M C30770; National Coordinating Center for the Regional GeneticsNetworks).

may provide more age-appropriate information and decrease other confounding factors.

Blood transfusions can confound certain testing on the newborn screening, including the hemoglobinopathies and the tests that rely on measuring enzyme activity (biotinidase, galactosemia). If a baby has had a transfusion prior to the newborn screen, the screen will have to be repeated at a time in which the blood products will no longer complicate the results.

Some analytes on the newborn screen can reflect maternal conditions rather than a disorder in the baby. With some disorders, mothers are tested in conjunction with their newborn to figure out who is truly affected.[25]

The future of newborn screening

Newborn screening continues to expand as additional disorders are being nominated to be included. To be included on the RUSP, an advisory committee must carefully consider the natural history of the disorder, the efficacy and availability of treatment, the screening methods and more. In recent years there has been a huge increase in the available treatments for genetic diseases, including things such as targeted medications, enzyme replacement therapy, and gene therapy. As efficacious treatments become available, more and more disorders become potential targets for screening.[26]

There has also been much discussion on further expanding newborn screening in the future to potentially include large-scale genomic sequencing. Multiple studies performing whole exome or whole genome sequencing on dried blood spots have been performed. However, sensitivity and specificity of whole exome sequencing has been found to be less than traditional newborn screening methods such as tandem mass spectrometry. Besides accuracy, there are other issues that would need to be resolved including turn around time and cost. The use of WES as a second-tier test has been suggested to help reduce false positives and potentially reduce the time to final diagnosis.[27]

With the advent of new technology and new treatment options, newborn screening has the potential to change much more rapidly than before. Pediatricians must remain up to date on the disorders being screened for in their state, to ensure they are equipped to provide appropriate follow-up and referrals if needed.

SUMMARY

Newborn screening is a vital public health service that prevents much morbidity and mortality in infants and children. The RUSP provides guidance to states on what disorders should be screened for, although there may be some variability between states on the disorders tested and how they are screened for. Because newborn screening is just a screen, and there can be many confounding factors, confirmatory testing must be done on all positives to confirm the diagnosis. On the other hand, providers must remember disorders can be missed on newborn screening as well, and keep these conditions in their differential diagnosis when presented with a child with concerning symptoms. Newborn screening continues to expand due to new treatment availability for rare diseases, a better understanding of these conditions and new technologies allowing for wide-scale screening. It is important for pediatricians to be aware of what is on the newborn screen, and how to appropriately follow up on a positive screen.

DISCLOSURE

Nothing to disclose.

REFERENCES

1. Wroblewska-Seniuk KE, Dabrowski P, Szyfter W, et al. Universal newborn hearing screening: methods and results, obstacles, and benefits. Pediatr Res 2017;81(3): 415–22.
2. Jullen S. Newborn pulse oximetry screening for critical congenital heart defects. BMC Pediatr 2021;21(1):305.
3. Martin GR, Ewer AK, Gaviglio A. Updated Strategies for Pulse Oximetry Screening for Critical Congenital Heart Disease. Pediatrics 2020;146(1):1–10.
4. Hoppe CC. Prenatal and newborn screening for hemoglobinopathies. Int. Jnl. Lab. Hem. 2013;35:297–305.
5. Meier ER. Treatment Options for Sickle Cell Disease. Pediatr Clin North Am 2018; 65(3):427–44.
6. Ali S, Mumtaz S, Shakir HA, et al. Current status of beta-thalassemia and it's treatment strategies. Mol Genet Genomic Med 2021;9:1–14.
7. Rastogi MV, LaFranchi SH. Congenital Hypothyroidism. Orphanet J Rare Dis 2010;5(17):1–22.
8. Pass KA, Neto EC. Update: Newborn screening for Endocrinopathies. Endocrinol Metab Clin N Am 2009;38(4):827–37.
9. Speiser PW, Arlt W, Auchus RJ. Congenital Adrenal Hyperplasia Due to Steroid 21-Hydoxylase Deficiency: An Endocrine Society Clinical Practice Guideline. J Clin Endocrinol Metab 2018;103(11):4043–88.
10. King JR, Hammarstrom L. Newborn Screening for Primary Immunodeficiency Diseases: History, Current and Future Practices. J Clin Immuno 2018;38:56–66.
11. Chinn IK, Shearer WT. Severe Combined Immunodeficiency Disorders. Immunol Allergy Clin North Am 2015;35(4):671–94.
12. Dickinson KM, Callaco JM. Cystic Fibrosis. Pediatr Rev 2021;42(2):55–67.
13. Rosenfeld M, Sontag MK, Ren CL. Cystic Fibrosis Diagnosis and Newborn Screening. Pediatr Clin N Am 2016;63:599–615.
14. McCandless SE, Wright EJ. Mandatory newborn screening in the United States: History, current status, and existential challenges. Birth Defects Research 2020; 112:350–66.
15. Sklirou E, Lichter-Koneck U. Inborn Errors of Metabolism with Cognitive Impairment: Metabolism Defects of Phenylalanine, Homocysteine and Methionine, Purine, and Pyrimidine, and Creatine. Pediatr Clin N Am 2018;65:267–77.
16. Schillaci LP, DeBrosse SD, McCandless SE. Inborn Errors of Metabolism with Acidosis: Organic Acidemias and Defects of Pyruvate and Ketone Body Metabolism. Pediatr Clin N Am 2018;65:209–30.
17. Summar ML, Mew NA. Inborn Errors of Metabolism with Hyperammonemia: Urea Cycle Defects and Related Disorders. Pediatr Clin N Am 2018;65(2):231–46.
18. El-Gharbawy A, Vockley J. Defects of Fatty Acid Oxidation and the Carnitine Shuttle System. Pediatr Clin N Am 2018;65(2):317–35.
19. Demirbas D, Brucker WJ, Berry GT. Inborn Errors of Metabolism with Hepatopathy: Metabolism Defects of Galactose, Fructose, and Tyrosine. Pediatr Clin N Am 2018;65(2):337–52.
20. Peake RWA, Bodamer OA. Newborn Screening for Lysosomal Storage Disorders. J Pediatr Genet 2017;6:51–60.
21. Zhu J, Eichler F, Biffi A. The Changing Face of Adrenoleukodystrophy. Endo Rev 2020;41(4):577–93.

22. Hale K, Ojodu J, Singh S. Landscape of Spinal Muscular Atrophy Newborn Screening in the United States: 2018-2021. Int. J. Neonatal Screen. 2021; 7(33):1–10.
23. Schorling DC, Pechmann A, Kirschner J. Advances in Treatment of Spinal Muscular Atrophy - New Phenotypes, New Challenges, New Implications for Care. J Neuromuscul Dis 2020;7(1):1–13.
24. Newborn Screening Timeliness Goals. Health Resources & Services Administration. Updated September 2017. Available at: https://www.hrsa.gov/advisory-committees/heritable-disorders/newborn-screening-timeliness. Accessed October 27, 2022.
25. El-Hattab AW, Almannai M, Sutton VR. Newborn Screening: History, Current Status, and Future Directions. Pediatr Clin North Am 2018;65(2):389–405.
26. Rajabi F. Updates in Newborn Screening. Pediatr Annals 2018;47(5):e187–90.
27. Adhikari AN, Gallagher RC, Wang T, et al. The Role of Exome Sequencing in Newborn Screening for Inborn Errors of Metabolism. Nat Med 2020;26(9):1392–7.

Ethical Aspects of Pediatric Genetic Care

Testing and Treatment

Kelly E. Ormond, MS, CGC[a,b,*], Alessandro Blasimme, PhD[a],
Effy Vayena, PhD[a]

KEYWORDS

- Ethics • Autonomy • Future interests of the child • Best interests
- Surrogate decision making

KEY POINTS

- Genetic testing in children requires the identification of an appropriate surrogate decision maker, and considerations about the value of relevant information for the biological relatives of the child.
- Predictive genetic tests, particularly those with typically adult onset, should be evaluated carefully in the consideration of the future autonomy interests of the child. Professional guidelines are available.
- Caring for children with genetic diseases raises ethical issues beyond simply genetic testing; additional clinical care issues may include treatment decisions, goals of care, and end-of-life care, as well as just access to available care options.

INTRODUCTION

Genetic and genomic testing has expanded dramatically since 2010. Pediatricians, both in general pediatric practice and in various pediatric specialties, will encounter diagnostic and predictive genetic screening and testing and the subsequent cascade testing that follows a new diagnosis, gene-based treatments (such as gene therapy, somatic gene editing, and molecular gene silencing treatments), and will support parents learning about and adapting to new diagnoses and difficult prognoses for their current (and potentially future) children. In this article, we review some of the ethical issues specific to pediatric medical care, with a focus on those that arise in the context of providing genetic care to children and their families.

[a] Department of Health Sciences and Technology, Health Ethics & Policy Lab, ETH Zurich. Hottingerstrasse 10, Zurich 8092, Switzerland; [b] Department of Genetics and Stanford Center for Biomedical Ethics, Stanford University School of Medicine
* Corresponding author. Department of Health Sciences and Technology, Health Ethics & Policy Lab, ETH Zurich. Hottingerstrasse 10, Zurich 8092, Switzerland.
E-mail address: kelly.ormond@hest.ethz.ch

Pediatr Clin N Am 70 (2023) 1029–1046
https://doi.org/10.1016/j.pcl.2023.05.011
0031-3955/23/© 2023 Elsevier Inc. All rights reserved.

Ethical issues (or ELSI, which stands for ethical, legal, and social issues) are frequently discussed when talking about genetics and genomics. This likely derives from several things. First, the history of eugenics. Second, genetics is inherently a family affair - not only do genetic conditions also indicate potential risk to other family members, but genetic testing can inadvertently discover information that identifies family members or information about the family structure. It also raises the question of whether it is ethically permissible to perform pediatric genetic testing primarily for family benefit. Genetic information can be diagnostic or predictive and probabilistic, depending on the timing and type of testing that is performed. The uncertainty and future predictability of this sort of information is not entirely novel to genetics, but in pediatrics it raises issues around the future autonomy of a child in deciding whether they do or do not want to know it. Genetic information, and our potential to change it, also raises discussion about what it means to be human and how our genes relate to our identity. And finally, genetic and genomic testing and treatments often blur the lines between clinically accepted treatments and research offerings. The rich history of ELSI research in the United States is nicely reviewed by Dolan et al (2022).[1]

Most pediatricians and pediatric health care providers will have taken a course in medical ethics during their training, and as a result will be familiar with a "Principles based approach" to ethics.[2] *Autonomy* references the importance of respecting individual persons, and is often enacted through informed consent. *Beneficence* references the importance of "doing good" and providing benefit to patients through our medical care or research, and *nonmaleficence* is the Hippocratic principle of "do no harm" and minimizing risks. Finally, the principle of *justice* argues for equity in access, and often reflects issues such as access issues, cost and insurance coverage, and accessibility across different populations (eg, ancestral backgrounds, LGBTQ+, sex). These principles are applicable in both a clinical setting and research setting, and in fact these principles underlie much of research ethics in the United States as they informed the Belmont Report.[3] Many other ethics approaches exist, including virtue ethics, which focuses on the importance of the conduct of the person, and gives guidance toward what virtuous or "right" actions might be. For example, veracity (truthtelling), or fidelity (trustworthiness) or transparency (which also comes up in conflict of interest issues) might be described as virtuous actions. To use veracity as an example, this ethical principle may arise when providing difficult prognostic information to parents (for example, breaking the news about a fatal diagnosis), when telling children the truth about their health or about inherited genetic risks, and when clinicians are asked to withhold information (or even lie) from children or adolescents.

Having now discussed many of the foundational ELSI issues around genetic testing in children, we will present some case examples to elaborate on additional ethical issues that may arise. When considering one's own practice and evaluating the ethical issues that may be in tension, there are many approaches that one might consider to standardize the process. Key across all the approaches are to (1) identify the potential ethical issues, (2) identify the range of options, (3) determine the relevant patient/family values, and (4) determine the course of action in consultation with the family. In ethics, there is not a "formula" for how to resolve ethical conflicts - no single principle or ethical framework trumps all others. Context is important, and the ethical frameworks that exist primarily provide clinicians with ways to think through the conflict, identifying which issues are important and why. Many times, ethics frameworks will reach the same conclusion based on the factors that are considered. The goal of this article is not to turn readers into clinical ethics consultants, but rather to sensitize pediatric care providers to the relevant ELSI issues that arise when providing genetic care, and to help them identify potential issues, the relevant professional guidelines that exist, and when cases may benefit from referrals and/or ethics consultation.

COMMON ETHICAL ISSUES IN PEDIATRIC GENETICS

Pediatric medical care raises the issue of surrogate decision making, which becomes even more complex when we add the importance of preserving the future autonomy of the child ("an open future"), the role of identity (particularly around treatment decisions or discussions around treatments that could be considered enhancement), and the potential for future identifiability and privacy issues. While we will not discuss them in detail, ethical issues that cross all areas of genetic testing and care include transparency about the uncertainty and changeability in variant interpretation, as well as about the potential use of AI and machine learning in variant interpretation, social justice, and equity issues that arise due to the fact that currently the majority of genetic data comes from persons of primarily white European ancestry, and issues related to the cost and accessibility of genetic testing and treatments.

Applying Autonomy to Genetic Testing Decisions: Informed Consent

As with any other medical procedure, the process of informed consent is critical to ensuring respect for persons and their autonomy. In general, informed consent means that a person is free to make a decision without coercion and that they can comprehend the risks and benefits of their medical options, and voice a choice. When evaluating the potential risks and benefits with genetic testing in general, it is important for health care providers to remember that unlike many medical procedures where the primary risks are physical risks, in genetic testing these risks are usually minimal (usually a blood draw or buccal swab), while the social and psychological risks may be more impactful. For example, some genetic tests pose a chance that unexpected family relationships could be discovered, as could an unexpected diagnosis (either incidentally or as part of a secondary findings analysis). Others may pose psychological risks such as anxiety or depression (for example a predictive test for a condition that has no medical treatments to change its course). And still others may pose risks to privacy or for discrimination, or that covered services may change with a diagnosis (for example in a school setting, or therapies). When considering benefits, clinical utility (medical actionability through screening or treatment) is also not the only potential benefit. Many individuals and families find personal utility in genetic testing[4]; for example, finding a genetic cause for current symptoms can relieve parental guilt that they somehow caused the condition through actions in pregnancy or early childhood, a predictive diagnosis can allow for research moving into the future, as well as potential lifestyle changes that may improve morbidity and long term mortality risks (for example, avoiding starting to smoke as a teen). Even when genetic test results are positive, the reduction in anxiety that arises from uncertainty can be helpful, and may allow adolescents and young adults to plan their future lives (eg, schooling, career, and family planning) in a more informed manner.[5–7] A recent systematic review suggests that at least for genomic sequencing, parents struggle to understand and recall relevant components of informed consent,[8] particularly around privacy and potential discrimination, future use of data beyond the clinical purposes, and secondary findings. This suggests that providers should simplify relevant principles, utilize appropriate health literacy-based communication strategies, and refer to skilled genetics providers when possible.[9]

The Special Case of Medical Decision Making for Children: Developing Autonomy and Interests for "an Open Future"

When discussing medical decision making in *pediatric* genetic care, we must also start by thinking about decision making capacity and the promotion of the autonomy of the child. In most countries, children do not have legal competence until age 18 or the age of the majority, though this varies slightly by country. Some countries and states also have specific regulations that allow children to make some medical decisions prior to reaching that age of majority (for example, emancipated minors; see the UN Convention of the Rights of the Child, 1989[10]). However, there is general appreciation that children develop decision making capacity over time, and as such, most children older than age 7 are asked to assent or dissent to medical procedures (including genetic testing), and as they become adolescents and young adults they should be increasingly actively included in the decision making process. Each health care provider should be familiar with the laws and regulations in their location of practice.[11,12] In most locations, the parent or guardian is considered the legal decision maker for children, and because children do not typically have enough lived experience for them to make surrogate decisions based on previously expressed values and wishes, most decision making follows the "best interest standard." The best interest standard assumes that parents and guardians generally know the child best, and will make decisions that will benefit the child and family. There is typically a lot of latitude granted to parents as long as the medical choices are not seen as being harmful or neglectful of the child.[11,12]

Beyond the traditional issues that surround pediatric decision making, genetics raises a new set of issues that relate to the autonomy of the child under care. While some genetic testing occurs symptomatically, and provides a diagnosis that explains a constellation of symptoms currently experienced by a child (eg, a karyotype or array CGH to explain intellectual disability, or an exome or genome sequence performed on a child suspected of having a genetic condition), even these diagnostic tests can lead to unexpected findings - whether about a family relationship or about an unexpected diagnosis. Beyond these diagnostic tests, a large percentage of genetic testing is predictive. For example, an exome test might identify a genetic variant that causes illness in late childhood, but it may also identify a variant associated only with adult-onset symptoms. These conditions may also have variable penetrance, variable expressivity and variable ages of onset, and may or may not have medical actionability. And finally, stored genetic material (and even stored genetic data) can pose potential privacy risks down the line.

A topic that has arisen often in the discussion about pediatric predictive genetic testing is often referred to as the right (or interest) that children have in an open future. This principle was first expounded in 1980,[13] with applications to genetic testing soon in the 1990s (eg, work by Dena Davis). Broadly, this concept suggests that while parents can generally raise their children based on their own values, there may be some key life choices that may have irreversible impact, and the child has a "right" (or, as per Garrett and colleagues, 2019, an interest) in keeping their options open, thus saving the option for them to exercise their future autonomy. A child's right to an open future is a right in trust, that is "to be *saved* for the child until he is an adult, but which can be violated "in advance," so to speak, before the child is even in a position to exercise [it]. His right while he is still a child is to have these future options kept open until he is a fully formed self-determining adult capable of deciding among them."[14] Testing children for adult-onset conditions, particularly for those which no treatment exists (eg, Huntington disease), would deprive the child of the possibility of deciding whether to undertake a test later on in his or her life while not offering any medical benefit. Many have argued however that knowing in advance about such conditions may indeed be important for the child and the family alike in terms of advanced planning. Garrett and colleagues (2019) argue that this is best understood not as a right but as an *interest*, which provides flexibility to balance future interests against other benefits and harms, as compared to a *right*, which would generate a duty on the parents (and potentially health care professionals) to strictly avoid pediatric predictive genetic testing.

Because of the many types of genetic testing that exist and the complexity of these issues, genetics societies across the world have created guidance about genetic testing in children, frequently centering around preserving the future interests of children to decide whether or not they wish to learn their genetic information,[15] and around the premise of reducing potential harms. We have summarized many of these guidelines in **Table 1**, though this is not an all-inclusive list of guidelines.

Reviewers of this table will note that all the professional societies support diagnostic testing, with some suggesting that clinicians order the most "narrow" test so as to minimize the chances of unexpected findings. This includes diagnostic genetic tests including for children who are being considered for adoption, even if they do not have medical treatments available. It is worth noting these recommendations preceded some organizations recommending exome or genome sequencing as a first-line diagnostic test, and that generally these tests are considered acceptable on the basis that the potential benefits (treatments, prognostic knowledge) outweigh potential harms in the face of symptoms. As one moves across the table, tests which provide less immediate clinical or personal utility are less supported. For example, testing for conditions that occur in childhood, even if not yet presenting symptomatically, are considered acceptable by most professional organizations. However, as conditions have later onset (eg, in adulthood, including carrier testing) they become less supported, with most organizations suggesting either complete deferral of these tests or, in specific situations where an adolescent and family are in agreement about their desire for testing, ensuring that a rigorous consent process is undergone. Importantly, most of the recommendations to defer predictive testing into adulthood are based on normative concerns for harm[16]; several also add reminders that even if testing is deferred, there can be significant benefit to communicating about genetic risk and future testing options to children (eg,[17]). There is limited empiric data about the actual harms when testing is performed[18,19]; most of the information about predictive testing centers around carrier testing,[7,20–22] familial adenometous polyposis (FAP) testing[23,24] and BRCA testing.[25] There is also a growing body of literature to suggest that young adults desire information sooner than it is given to them by their parents, and that an open communication approach about genetic risk status in the family is beneficial ([26,27]). As a result of this empiric data, over time many of the genetic society guidelines have become more flexible about the potential consideration of predictive genetic testing for adolescents, reflecting what had been happening in practice over time (for example,[28,29]). It is important to consider the developmental stages of childhood and adolescence when contemplating genetic testing of children[30]; several authors have also proposed conceptual frameworks for sharing genetic risk information, genetic counseling, and consideration of genetic testing in children.[31–33]

The Issues of Unsolicited Findings

The expansion of genetic testing toward genomic testing has raised the issue of unsolicited findings in the past 10+ years. These findings are sometimes referred to as incidental findings (by which we will refer to findings that are unexpected and not searched for) and secondary findings (by which we will refer to findings that are

Table 1
Summary of international guidelines on genetic testing in children (as of 2022)

Type of genetic Test/Professional group	Predictive, Childhood, Treatable	Predictive, Childhood, not Treatable	Predictive, Adult	Incidental or Secondary Findings (Adult)	Carrier Screen	Adoption (Symptomatic and predictive Testing)	Direct to Consumer
AAP/ACMG 2013 (USA)	Yes	Yes	Defer (flexibility)	Refer to Miller et al., 2021. Offer regardless of age.	No, unless pregnant	Consistent with general recommendations for any child	Strongly discourage
ASHG 2015 (USA)	Yes	Not overtly discussed	Defer (flexibility)	Optional, with strong consent process.	Neutral	Consistent with general recommendations for any child	Discourage
Canadian Pediatric Society	Yes		Defer	Refer to Boycott et al. 2015.	Discuss	Consistent with general recommendations for any child	Strongly discourage
ESHG 2009 (EU)	Yes	Optional	Defer unless early actions possible	See deWert et al. 2021 - recommend avoid opportunistic screening	Discourage	Not overtly discussed	Not overtly discussed
BSMG 2022 (UK)	Yes. Special notes re: cardiac testing	Yes	Defer (flexibility)	No consensus. Refer to deWert et al. 2021	Defer (flexibility)	Consistent with general recommendations for any child	Not overtly discussed
HGSA 2020 (Australia)	Yes	Discuss	Defer (flexiblity)	Not overtly discussed	Not overtly discussed	Not overtly discussed	Not overtly discussed

searched for but unrelated to the primary testing indication, such as genes included on the ACMG v3.0 secondary findings lists[34]; some literature also refers to this as "opportunistic screening"[35]) The return of incidental and secondary findings to children has been well debated in the literature, and the normative concerns primarily surround the feasibility to obtain informed consent (particularly when parents are focused on issues that surround the primary testing indication), and issues that mirror predictive testing in children and include privacy, discrimination, future autonomy, and emotional harms, particularly if a condition is not medically actionable for years. Some researchers also raise the potential family benefits that may accrue if a secondary finding is identified in a child, such that at risk parents could be identified and with the potential to decrease their morbidity or mortality.[36,37]

Shortly after genomic sequencing became available, studies assessed the hypothetical interest in receiving secondary findings.[38–41] More recently, adolescents and children enrolled in genomic research have also been studied with regards to their hypothetical and actual interest in return of results.[42–44] Importantly, some studies[45,46] have found that parents do not necessarily differentiate between primary and secondary results, but rather consider all to be potentially relevant health information. While parents were often interested in receiving predictive secondary findings, they may wait until adolescence to disclose the results to the child and there is emerging data that they found familial benefit to knowing about a hereditary risk.[45]

Expanding Towards Genomic Newborn Screening

Newborn screening (NBS) was initially based on principles developed by Wilson and Junger[47] and elaborated upon by Dobrow.[48] These principles generally suggest that NBS can be offered for asymptomatic infants if we have sufficient information about a health condition (including its natural history), an acceptable and effective test and treatment is available, and that the implementation of a screening program is feasible and cost-effective. The public health format of newborn screening means that is offered universally, and that it also involves a more limited consent model (in some cases, an "opt-out" approach, where a parent must actively decline newborn screening, rather than consenting to have their child undergo it). This near universality of NBS combined with the loss of parental autonomy require that the included conditions are well justified with regards to their seriousness, urgency, and treatability.[49]

In the early 2000s, newborn screening began to expand from the traditionally included conditions such as phenylketonuria (PKU) to a much wider list of conditions, including some (eg, Krabbe, Pompe and X-linked adrenoleukodystrophy, X-ALD) that were controversial for their later childhood onset, significant phenotypic variability and limited treatment options.[49] The potential inclusion of these conditions raised public health ethics concerns that focused on the potential increase in harm and decrease in beneficial outcomes, raised ethical questions about how conditions are chosen for inclusion on NBS panels. For example, how is benefit for a public health screening tool assessed when you move beyond clinical utility into personal utility and family benefits? Also, who should determine which conditions are included?[49,50] Over time in both in the United States and Europe this NBS expansion has happened inconsistently and despite the existence of a Recommended Uniform Screening Panel in the US, primarily since policy decisions about newborn screening being made on a state-by-state or country-by-country basis respectively.[51–53] This consequent variability in screening approaches raises the important ethical issue of equity and access. Finally, one last ethical issue haunts newborn screening: in recent years there have been privacy concerns about the re-use of dried blood spots without parental permission.[54] Since these blood spots contain DNA, and are inherently identifiable, there are worries about privacy violations, potential discrimination, and familial implications.

In recent years, genomic screening of neonates is becoming increasingly realistic (https://www.genome.gov/Funded-Programs-Projects/Newborn-Sequencing-in-Genomic-Medicine-and-Public-Health-NSIGHT, accessed 8 Nov 2022). Some of these genomic approaches use a focused approach (eg, a targeted gene panel), while others use an exome or genomic sequencing approach that could analyze and report on any potential genes. Neonatal genomic approaches raise similar issues to those already discussed in pediatric screening: how to obtain appropriate consent, the selection of the conditions returned, particularly if they are later childhood or adult onset, the balance of benefits and harms, and the equity issues that will arise. There is an emerging body of knowledge available about the use of newborn genomic testing in sick neonates (eg, rapid sequencing in a NICU), as well as the potential to use genomic sequencing in healthy appearing neonates to predict a range of future illnesses.[55,56] Most professional organizations and ethics advisory panels (eg the NSIGHT EAB) have found that broadly offering genomic screening to healthy neonates is premature as the potential for harm outweighs the current potential for benefit[57–60] While there may be beneficence in the case of a new treatable diagnosis that would not otherwise be identified in standard NBS, the potential benefits (and often the interpretations and prospective meaning of the information) remain unclear. As was evidenced by the expanded NBS examples of Krabbe and Pompe disease, harm may occur through unnecessary interventions and long term monitoring, parental anxiety, and impact on the parent-child relationship.[61] And importantly the issues of how to achieve consent and cost implications on the public health system remain unanswered.

GENETICS AND THE FAMILY

Genetic testing impacts both the patient and the family. Typically in medicine, the "care unit" is considered to be the patient. But of course any clinician will recognize that medical decision-making impacts family members in a number of ways. With genetic testing, a new genetic diagnosis has implications on other family members who are at risk.

Case example 1: a genetic test is performed on a symptomatic child for cystic fibrosis, an autosomal recessive condition. The child has two identifiable pathogenic mutations; one of which is carried by the mother, but the other is not carried by the purported father, suggesting he is not the biological father of the child. What are the duties of the medical provider to disclose the relevant information, particularly that the couple is not at 25% risk in future pregnancies, and the "father" is not a carrier of CF.

Case example 2: A child is diagnosed with a genetic condition that is carried by a parent. The parent does not wish to disclose the genetic risk information to relatives who may also carry the mutation (eg, the child's aunts and uncles, who are also of reproductive age), putting their future children at potential risk. What are the duties of the medical provider to encourage sharing this genetic information? Are there any "duties to warn" these at-risk relatives?

Key ethical principles including privacy, veracity, beneficence, and nonmaleficence are important in evaluating these cases; the ethic of care and its focus on relationships is particularly relevant in cases that involve the family as a unit. In both cases, privacy and veracity are directly in conflict when a family member does not wish to divulge relevant genetic information. This potential lack of truthfulness impacts family members' ability to exercise their autonomy. However, these cases highlight several challenges when ethical principles may conflict. For example, in Case 1, potential approaches include (1) fully disclosing the information to both members of the couple, (2) privately disclosing to the mother with encouragement to disclose relevant details and assessing the situation, or (3) disclosing simply that they are not at elevated risk for having a future affected child. Full disclosure to the parents that misattributed parentage was present prioritizes veracity, but may pose a risk of harm to the family relationships, which could potentially lead to harm of the mother and/or child. However, a prospective parent may make reproductive decisions differently if informed accurately about their reproductive risks (or lack thereof). Options such as 3, which accurately discloses the couples risks but do not clarify that the putative father is not a carrier, withholds important information that his biologic offspring are not at risk to be affected (and that his siblings are not at increased risk above the population rate). Withholding this information may lead to unnecessary anxiety and future testing in some individuals. Professional societies provide different advice on how best to handle the conflicting obligations of privacy and veracity in the case of misattributed paternity. Here one might start by asking: Will the child's care change on the basis of disclosure? What are the potential harms on each person with each option of disclosure, and how likely are they to occur?[62] From there, one could weigh the impact on privacy, autonomy, and the ratio of beneficence and nonmaleficence.

Case 2 raises issues about disclosure to family members who are more distant and not part of the immediate family that is being tested. These family members will frequently not be patients of the care provider. How does the clinician handle the conflict of protecting the privacy of their patient, who has explicitly said they do not wish to share the information? Here again, one might ask: What is the condition under discussion, and what are the potential harms with and without disclosure? For example, is the condition highly penetrant and the relatives are at a high risk? Could they change the morbidity and mortality associated with the condition through screening or early identification? Are they likely to undergo routine testing or screening for this condition for other reasons (for example is it included on routine carrier screening panels)?

In the case of a family disclosure, the clear moral duty of the medical provider is to ensure that the relevant family member is provided with accurate information and encouraged to share the it with the at-risk family members, with some recent legal findings (ABC vs St Georges Health Care) suggesting there may be stronger legal duties to inform in some jurisdictions.[62–67] As in many ethically complex situations, often a combination of encouragement by the medical provider and time will resolve the situation and lead to the disclosure of important genetic information. Beyond this, the law in different countries varies regarding what the legal duties for informing relatives are even when a patient declines to do so themselves[68–71] These examples emphasize one final key point – given the chance that unexpected family relationships can be identified, and that pathogenic genetic testing results should be shared with at risk family members so they can consider cascade testing, these outcomes should be raised as part of the informed consent discussions *prior* to genetic testing so that the patient or their parent is aware of the possibilities in advance.

TREATMENTS FOR GENETIC DISEASE

While genetic disease has always had symptomatic treatment approaches, there are increasingly new approaches that may lead to significant changes in morbidity and mortality for those with genetic conditions. Koogler and colleagues (2003) thoughtfully reviews the historical examples of treatment being withheld or withdrawn from children with genetic conditions (for example, a child with Down syndrome being denied heart surgery) and the underlying ethical issues that these situations raise.[72] Despite changes, parents still report challenges in obtaining health care for their children with genetic disease (eg,[73,74]).

Increasingly, new treatments are being developed for genetic conditions - these include treatments that provide lacking enzymes or decrease substrate buildup (for example, a bone marrow transplant or stem cell transplant for an inborn error of metabolism), gene-focused treatments that silence or "turn on" genes by addressing genetic mechanisms such as splicing (eg, treatments for Duchenne muscular dystrophy or spinal muscular atrophy), or somatic gene therapies or gene editing approaches (eg, for sickle cell disease or specific forms of congenital blindness). Given the rare frequency of most genetic diseases, there can be a blur between research and clinical treatments, sometimes meaning that the only potential option for treatment is a clinical trial. They may also have quite invasive and potentially risky forms of administration. For example, Nusinersen is injected via lumbar puncture, requires frequent doses and has a cost into the millions of US dollars; it is just one example of the potential harms that are associated with the treatment of rare disease.[75] Once safety testing is complete and regulatory approvals are obtained, treatments may become expensive or limited to specific high-level hospitals, both of which limit potential access to the treatments. In recent years, there has been a shift from discussions about these potential harms (including potential death, stemming from the death of Jesse Gelsinger in early gene therapy trials), to excessive hope that the therapy will be a disease cure.[76] From the perspective of justice, is it ethically appropriate to offer treatments that are realistically only available to a small segment of the population that may need them? In countries that provide nationally funded health care systems, what are the ethical issues in choosing to pay for these rare but extremely expensive treatments when it takes away health care dollars from other sick persons? How do we balance these public health funding issues?[77]

Recent technical advances in gene and cell therapy hold great promise to tackle numerous conditions, including hereditary ones. A number of clinical trials are underway regarding innovative regenerative medicine treatments with the potential to address a variety of pediatric conditions that have a genetic component. Such trials usually have very strict inclusion criteria and are open to very few patients. Family and caretakers may rightly see trial enrollment as a concrete chance of accessing a potentially beneficial treatment. It is thus important that enrollment decisions are fully transparent and inspired by ethically robust criteria and decisional mechanisms. As a result of the extremely limited opportunities to enroll in innovative clinical trials, many families may be tempted to obtain yet unproven treatments, often offered abroad, in countries with insufficient safeguards and regulatory standards.[78,79]

Finally, while many people focus on the issues of safety and cost for somatic gene-based therapies, they also raise important issues around identity and issues such as support and stigma that center around the social model of disability.[80] In contrast to the medical model of disability, which assumes that a genetic condition impairs quality of life and should be corrected when possible, the social model of disability suggests that the impairments that occur due to chronic illness are socially based. Extending the expressionist argument beyond prenatal testing,[81] one might imagine that decreasing the number of people impacted by a genetic condition might decrease social support, and also lead to stigma when an individual or family chose not to undergo a specific treatment. There are also a growing number of studies that suggest that people with genetic illness and their families have differing, and sometimes quite nuanced, views toward gene editing and gene therapies as treatments for their condition.[82–86]

END-OF-LIFE ISSUES FOR A CHILD WITH A GENETIC CONDITION

Genetic conditions have a higher mortality rate, and are in fact responsible for a substantial percentage of neonatal intensive care unit (NICU) stays and neonatal and early childhood deaths.[87] As such, pediatricians caring for children with genetic disease will be faced with having hard conversations with parents about their child's prognosis, and to help them set goals of care toward the end of life that match their family values. Some studies suggest that rapid genomic sequencing in a NICU setting can help clarify a diagnosis and help guide these care decisions.[88–92]

End-of-life decision making is complex and emotionally challenging for patients of any age. In childhood, while the parents (or guardians) are the legal decision makers, children's autonomy should be respected to the degree that is appropriate for their age. Ethical principles such as veracity and autonomy are important here and could be respected by sharing age appropriate information with children about their health status and treatments, and including older children and adolescents in decision-making to the extent that it is appropriate.[93,94]

Ethical conflicts may arise with regards to disagreements between the parents, between parents and the child, or between the family and the medical team with regards to end-of-life care, particularly when it comes to withholding or withdrawing treatments. Major goals might include avoiding suffering (beneficence and nonmaleficience) and facilitating informed decisions (veracity about the prognosis and uncertainties, autonomy to make decisions based on personal values, and consideration of future quality of life issues).[95] Palliative care specialists and ethics consultants can often assist in navigating these complex discussions about goals of care and medical decision making at the end of life.

SUMMARY

There are many ethical issues that arise in caring for children and their families facing genetic disease. In considering genetic testing, one must consider the type of screening or testing being offered, the age of the child, and the larger context as it relates to the child's current and future interests. Professional guidelines can provide a health care provider with a starting place for discussion with the family, including the consideration of the interests in preserving the child's future autonomy for predictive genetic testing decisions. Any provider who is ordering genetic testing should identify the proper surrogate decision maker and involve the child in testing discussions and obtain assent as is developmentally appropriate. Beyond genetic testing, caring for families with genetic disease can raise issues of family disclosure, privacy, treatment decisions and end-of-life care.

CLINICS CARE POINTS

- Many professional organizations around the world have published guidelines regarding the use of genetic testing in childhood.
- Informed consent for genetic testing and considering of the developing autonomy of children is important, especially for predictive genetic tests and those that return secondary or incidental findings.

- Genetic testing results can raise complicated family issues, such as misattributed parentage and issues regarding sharing genetic test results to at risk family members. These should be mentioned as part of the informed consent process.
- Health care providers can consider ethical consultations when they feel unprepared to address ethical issues that arise in providing genetic care to children.

DISCLOSURE

Nothing to disclose.

REFERENCES

1. Dolan DD, Lee SSJ, Cho MK. Three decades of ethical, legal, and social implications research: Looking back to chart a path forward. Cell Genom. 2022;2(7). doi:10.1016/j.xgen.2022.100150.
2. Beauchamp TL, Childress JF. Principles of Biomedical Ethics. Oxford: Oxford University Press; 1979.
3. National Commission for the Protection of Human Subjects of Biomedical and Behavioral Research. *The Belmont Report: Ethical Principles and Guidelines for the Protection of Human Subjects of Research.* U.S. Department of Health and Human Services. ; 1979. Available at: https://www.hhs.gov/ohrp/regulations-and-policy/belmont-report/read-the-belmont-report/index.html.
4. Kohler JN, Turbitt E, Biesecker BB. Personal utility in genomic testing: a systematic literature review. Eur J Hum Genet 2017;25(6):662–8. https://doi.org/10.1038/ejhg.2017.10.
5. Levenseller BL, Soucier DJ, Miller Va, et al. Stakeholders' opinions on the implementation of pediatric whole exome sequencing: Implications for informed consent. J Genet Couns 2014;23:552–65. https://doi.org/10.1007/s10897-013-9626-y.
6. Sabatello M, Chen Y, Sanderson SC, et al. Increasing genomic literacy among adolescents. Genet Med 2019;21(4):994–1000. https://doi.org/10.1038/s41436-018-0275-2.
7. McConkie-Rosell A, Spiridigliozzi GA, Melvin E, et al. Living with genetic risk: effect on adolescent self-concept. Am J Med Genet C Semin Med Genet 2008; 148C(1):56–69. https://doi.org/10.1002/ajmg.c.30161.
8. Gereis J, Hetherington K, Ha L, et al. Parents' understanding of genome and exome sequencing for pediatric health conditions: a systematic review. Eur J Hum Genet 2022;30(11):1216–25. https://doi.org/10.1038/s41431-022-01170-2.
9. Ormond KE, Hallquist MLG, Buchanan AH, et al. Developing a conceptual, reproducible, rubric-based approach to consent and result disclosure for genetic testing by clinicians with minimal genetics background. Genet Med 2018. https://doi.org/10.1038/s41436-018-0093-6.
10. Consenting to medical treatment without parental consent. European Union Agency for Fundamental Rights. Published November 14, 2017. Accessed November 10, 2022. Available at: https://fra.europa.eu/en/publication/2017/mapping-minimum-age-requirements-concerning-rights-child-eu/consenting-medical-treatment-without-parental-consent.
11. Weithorn LA. When Does A Minor's Legal Competence To Make Health Care Decisions Matter? Pediatrics 2020;146(Suppl 1):S25–32. https://doi.org/10.1542/peds.2020-0818G.

12. COMMITTEE ON BIOETHICS. Informed Consent in Decision-Making in Pediatric Practice. Pediatrics 2016;138(2). https://doi.org/10.1542/peds.2016-1484.
13. Feinberg J. CHAPTER THREE The Child's Right to an Open Future (1980). In: Freedom and Fulfillment. Princeton University Press; 2021:76-97. Accessed September 30, 2022. Available at: https://www.degruyter.com/document/doi/10.1515/9780691218144-005/html?lang=en.
14. Feinberg J. The child's right to an open future. In: Engster DMT, editor. Justice, Politics, and the family. 2015. p. 145–60.
15. Garrett JR, Lantos JD, Biesecker LG, et al. Rethinking the "open future" argument against predictive genetic testing of children. Genet Med 2019;21(10):2190–8. https://doi.org/10.1038/s41436-019-0483-4.
16. Mand C, Gillam L, Delatycki MB, et al. Predictive genetic testing in minors for late-onset conditions: a chronological and analytical review of the ethical arguments. J Med Ethics 2012;38:519–24. https://doi.org/10.1136/medethics-2011-100055.
17. Royal College of Physicians (RCP), Royal College of Pathologists (RCPath) and British Society for Genetic Medicine. (BSGM. Genetic testing in childhood. Guidance for clinical practice. Report of the Joint Committee on Genomics in Medicine. In: ; 2022.
18. Borry P, Stultiens L, Nys H, et al. Presymptomatic and predictive genetic testing in minors: a systematic review of guidelines and position papers. Clin Genet 2006; 70(5):374–81. https://doi.org/10.1111/j.1399-0004.2006.00692.x.
19. Wade CH, Wilfond BS, McBride CM. Effects of genetic risk information on children's psychosocial wellbeing: a systematic review of the literature. Genet Med 2010;12(X):317–26. https://doi.org/10.1097/GIM.0b013e3181de695c.
20. Järvinen O, Hietala M, Aalto AM, et al. A retrospective study of long-term psychosocial consequences and satisfaction after carrier testing in childhood in an autosomal recessive disease: aspartylglucosaminuria. Clin Genet 2000;58(6):447–54. https://doi.org/10.1034/j.1399-0004.2000.580604.x.
21. Järvinen O, Lehesjoki AE, Lindlöf M, et al. Carrier testing of children for two X-linked diseases: A retrospective study of comprehension of the test results and social and psychological significance of the testing. Pediatrics 2000; 106(6):1460–5. https://doi.org/10.1542/peds.106.6.1460.
22. McConkie-Rosell A, Spiridigliozzi GA, Sullivan JA, et al. Longitudinal study of the carrier testing process for fragile X syndrome: Perceptions and coping. Am J Med Genet 2001;98:37–45. https://doi.org/10.1002/1096-8628(20010101)98:1<37::AID-AJMG1006>3.0.CO;2-O.
23. Michie S, Bobrow M, Marteau TM. Predictive genetic testing in children and adults: a study of emotional impact. J Med Genet 2001;38(8):519–26. https://www.ncbi.nlm.nih.gov/pubmed/11483640.
24. Codori AM, Zawacki KL, Petersen GM, et al. Genetic testing for hereditary colorectal cancer in children: long-term psychological effects. Am J Med Genet 2003; 116A:117–28. https://doi.org/10.1002/ajmg.a.10926.
25. Bradbury AR, Patrick-Miller L, Schwartz LA, et al. Psychosocial adjustment and perceived risk among adolescent girls from families with BRCA1/2 or breast cancer history. J Clin Oncol 2016;34(28):3409–16. https://doi.org/10.1200/JCO.2015.66.3450.
26. Holt K. What do we tell the children? Contrasting the disclosure choices of two HD families regarding risk status and predictive genetic testing. J Genet Couns 2006; 15(4):253–65. https://doi.org/10.1007/s10897-006-9021-z.
27. Stuttgen K, McCague A, Bollinger J, et al. Whether, when, and how to communicate genetic risk to minors: "I wanted more information but I think they were

scared I couldn"t handle it. J Genet Couns 2021;30(1):237–45. https://doi.org/10.1002/jgc4.1314.

28. Duncan RE, Savulescu J, Gillam L, et al. An international survey of predictive genetic testing in children for adult onset conditions. Genet Med 2005;7(6):390–6. https://doi.org/10.1097/01.gim.0000170775.39092.44.

29. Fenwick A, Plantinga M, Dheensa S, et al. Predictive Genetic Testing of Children for Adult-Onset Conditions: Negotiating Requests with Parents. J Genet Couns 2017;26(2):244–50. https://doi.org/10.1007/s10897-016-0018-y.

30. Fanos JH. Developmental tasks of childhood and adolescence: Implications for genetic testing. Am J Med Genet 1997;71:22–8.

31. Mcconkie-rosell A, Spiridigliozzi GA. Family Matters ": A Conceptual Framework for Genetic Testing in. Children 2004;13(1):9–29.

32. Young MA, Thompson K, Lewin J, et al. A framework for youth-friendly genetic counseling. J Community Genet 2020;11(2):161–70. https://doi.org/10.1007/s12687-019-00439-2.

33. Werner-Lin A, Merrill SL, Brandt AC, et al. Talking with Children About Adult-Onset Hereditary Cancer Risk: A Developmental Approach for Parents. J Genet Couns 2018;27(3):533–48. https://doi.org/10.1007/s10897-017-0191-7.

34. Miller DT, Lee K, Chung WK, et al. ACMG SF v3.0 list for reporting of secondary findings in clinical exome and genome sequencing: a policy statement of the American College of Medical Genetics and Genomics (ACMG). Genet Med 2021;23(8):1381–90. https://doi.org/10.1038/s41436-021-01172-3.

35. de Wert G, Dondorp W, Clarke A, et al. Opportunistic genomic screening. Recommendations of the European Society of Human Genetics. Eur J Hum Genet 2021;29(3):365–77. https://doi.org/10.1038/s41431-020-00758-w.

36. Vayena E, Tasioulas J. Genetic incidental findings: autonomy regained? Genet Med 2013;15(11):868–70. https://doi.org/10.1038/gim.2013.104.

37. Wilfond BS, Fernandez CV, Green RC. Disclosing Secondary Findings from Pediatric Sequencing to Families: Considering the "Benefit to Families. J Law Med Ethics 2015;43(3):552–8. https://doi.org/10.1111/jlme.12298.

38. Shahmirzadi L, Chao EC, Palmaer E, et al. Patient decisions for disclosure of secondary findings among the first 200 individuals undergoing clinical diagnostic exome sequencing. Genet Med 2014;16(5):395–9. https://doi.org/10.1038/gim.2013.153.

39. Sapp JC, Dong D, Stark C, et al. Parental attitudes, values, and beliefs toward the return of results from exome sequencing in children. Clin Genet 2014;85:120–6. https://doi.org/10.1111/cge.12254.

40. Kleiderman E, Knoppers BM, Fernandez CV, et al. Returning incidental findings from genetic research to children: views of parents of children affected by rare diseases. J Med Ethics 2013;0:1–6. https://doi.org/10.1136/medethics-2013-101648.

41. Oberg JA, Glade Bender JL, Cohn EG, et al. Overcoming challenges to meaningful informed consent for whole genome sequencing in pediatric cancer research. Pediatr Blood Cancer 2015;62(8):1374–80. https://doi.org/10.1002/pbc.25520.

42. Pervola J, Myers MF, McGowan ML, et al. Giving adolescents a voice: the types of genetic information adolescents choose to learn and why. Genet Med 2019;21(4):965–71. https://doi.org/10.1038/s41436-018-0320-1.

43. Kulchak Rahm A, Bailey L, Fultz K, et al. Parental attitudes and expectations towards receiving genomic test results in healthy children. Transl Behav Med 2018;8(1):44–53. https://doi.org/10.1093/tbm/ibx044.

44. Savatt JM, Wagner JK, Joffe S, et al. Pediatric reporting of genomic results study (PROGRESS): a mixed-methods, longitudinal, observational cohort study protocol to explore disclosure of actionable adult- and pediatric-onset genomic variants to minors and their parents. BMC Pediatr 2020;20(1):222. https://doi.org/10.1186/s12887-020-02070-4.

45. Miner SA, Similuk M, Jamal L, et al. Genomic tools for health: Secondary findings as findings to be shared. Genet Med 2022. https://doi.org/10.1016/j.gim.2022.07.015.

46. Bowling KM, Thompson ML, Kelly MA, et al. Return of non-ACMG recommended incidental genetic findings to pediatric patients: considerations and opportunities from experiences in genomic sequencing. Genome Med 2022;14(1):131. https://doi.org/10.1186/s13073-022-01139-2.

47. Wilson JM, Jungner YG. Principles and practice of mass screening for disease. Bol Oficina Sanit Panam 1968;65(4):281–393. https://apps.who.int/iris/bitstream/handle/10665/37650/WHO_PHP_34.pdf?sequence=17.

48. Dobrow MJ, Hagens V, Chafe R, et al. Consolidated principles for screening based on a systematic review and consensus process. CMAJ (Can Med Assoc J) 2018;190(14):E422–9. https://doi.org/10.1503/cmaj.171154.

49. Currier RJ. Newborn Screening Is on a Collision Course with Public Health Ethics. Screening 2022;8(4). https://doi.org/10.3390/ijns8040051.

50. Petros M. Revisiting the Wilson-Jungner criteria: how can supplemental criteria guide public health in the era of genetic screening? Genet Med 2012;14(1):129–34. https://doi.org/10.1038/gim.0b013e31823331d0.

51. Watson MS, Lloyd-Puryear MA, Howell RR. The Progress and Future of US Newborn Screening. Screening 2022;8(3). https://doi.org/10.3390/ijns8030041.

52. Loeber JG, Platis D, Zetterström RH, et al. Neonatal Screening in Europe Revisited: An ISNS Perspective on the Current State and Developments Since 2010. Screening 2021;7(1). https://doi.org/10.3390/ijns7010015.

53. Sikonja J, Groselj U, Scarpa M, et al. Towards Achieving Equity and Innovation in Newborn Screening across Europe. Screening 2022;8(2). https://doi.org/10.3390/ijns8020031.

54. Hughes RIV, Choudhury S, Shah A. Newborn Screening Blood Spot Retention And Reuse: A Clash Of Public Health And Privacy Interests. Health Affairs Forefront 2022. https://doi.org/10.1377/forefront.20221004.177058.

55. Pereira S, Smith HS, Frankel LA, et al. Psychosocial Effect of Newborn Genomic Sequencing on Families in the BabySeq Project: A Randomized Clinical Trial. JAMA Pediatr 2021;175(11):1132–41. https://doi.org/10.1001/jamapediatrics.2021.2829.

56. Roman TS, Crowley SB, Roche MI, et al. Genomic Sequencing for Newborn Screening: Results of the NC NEXUS Project. Am J Hum Genet 2020;107(4):596–611. https://doi.org/10.1016/j.ajhg.2020.08.001.

57. Howard HC, Knoppers BM, Cornel MC, et al. Whole-genome sequencing in newborn screening? A statement on the continued importance of targeted approaches in newborn screening programmes. Eur J Hum Genet 2015;23(12):1593–600. https://doi.org/10.1038/ejhg.2014.289.

58. Johnston J, Lantos JD, Goldenberg A, et al. Sequencing Newborns: A Call for Nuanced Use of Genomic Technologies. Hastings Cent Rep 2018;48(Suppl 2):S2–6. https://doi.org/10.1002/hast.874.

59. The Ethics of Sequencing Newborns: Reflections and Recommendations - The Hastings Center. The Hastings Center. Published August 15, 2018. Accessed December 12, 2018. Available at: https://www.thehastingscenter.org/

publications-resources/special-reports-2/ethics-sequencing-newborns-reflections-recommendations/.

60. Kalkman, Dondorp. The case for screening in early life for "non-treatable"disorders: ethics, evidence and proportionality. A report from the Health Council of the Netherlands. Eur J Hum Genet 2022. Available at: https://www.nature.com/articles/s41431-022-01055-4.

61. Johnston J, Lantos JD, Goldenberg A, et al. Sequencing Newborns: A Call for Nuanced Use of Genomic Technologies. Hastings Cent Rep 2018;48(Suppl 2):S2–6.

62. Prero MY, Strenk M, Garrett J, et al. Disclosure of Misattributed Paternity. Pediatrics 2019;143(6). https://doi.org/10.1542/peds.2018-3899.

63. Carrieri D, Dheensa S, Doheny S, et al. Recontacting in clinical practice: an investigation of the views of healthcare professionals and clinical scientists in the United Kingdom. Eur J Hum Genet 2017;25(3):275–9. https://doi.org/10.1038/ejhg.2016.188.

64. Weaver M. The Double Helix: Applying an Ethic of Care to the Duty to Warn Genetic Relatives of Genetic Information. Bioethics 2016;30(3):181–7. https://doi.org/10.1111/bioe.12176.

65. Rothstein MA. Reconsidering the duty to warn genetically at-risk relatives. Genet Med 2018;20(3):285–90. https://doi.org/10.1038/gim.2017.257.

66. Foster C, Gilbar R. Is there a New Duty to Warn Family Members in English Medical Law? ABC V ST George's Healthcare NHS Trust and Others [2020] EWHC 4551. Med Law Rev 2021;29(2):359–72. https://doi.org/10.1093/medlaw/fwab006.

67. Anna M, Christine P, Jonathan R, et al. Professional duties are now considered legal duties of care within genomic medicine. Eur J Hum Genet 2020;28(10):1301–4. https://doi.org/10.1038/s41431-020-0663-3.

68. Phillips A, Bronselaer T, Borry P, et al. Informing relatives of their genetic risk: an examination of the Belgian legal context. Eur J Hum Genet 2022;30(7):766–71. https://doi.org/10.1038/s41431-021-01016-3.

69. de Paor A. Comment on Informing relatives of their genetic risk: an examination of the Belgian context. Eur J Hum Genet 2022;30(7):749–51. https://doi.org/10.1038/s41431-022-01066-1.

70. Meggiolaro N, Barlow-Stewart K, Dunlop K, et al. Disclosure to genetic relatives without consent - Australian genetic professionals' awareness of the health privacy law. BMC Med Ethics 2020;21(1):13. https://doi.org/10.1186/s12910-020-0451-1.

71. d'Audiffret Van Haecke D, de Montgolfier S. Genetic diseases and information to relatives: practical and ethical issues for professionals after introduction of a legal framework in France. Eur J Hum Genet 2018;26(6):786–95. https://doi.org/10.1038/s41431-018-0103-9.

72. Koogler TK, Wilfond BS, Ross LF. Lethal language, lethal decisions. Hastings Cent Rep 2003;33(2):37–41. https://doi.org/10.2307/3528153.

73. Morrison W. Please Let Me Hear My Son Cry Once. AMA Journal of Ethics 2010;12(7):530–4.

74. Feudtner C, Walter JK, Faerber JA, et al. Good-Parent Beliefs of Parents of Seriously Ill Children 2015;19104(1):39–47. https://doi.org/10.1001/jamapediatrics.2014.2341.

75. Burgart AM, Magnus D, Tabor HK, et al. Ethical Challenges Confronted When Providing Nusinersen Treatment for Spinal Muscular Atrophy. JAMA Pediatr 2018;172(2):188–92. https://doi.org/10.1001/jamapediatrics.2017.4409.

76. Broadfoot M. We Need to Ground Truth Assumptions about Gene Therapy. Nature 2021. https://doi.org/10.1038/d41586-021-02735-9.

77. Juth N, Henriksson M, Gustavsson E, et al. Should we accept a higher cost per health improvement for orphan drugs? A review and analysis of egalitarian arguments. Bioethics 2021;35(4):307–14. https://doi.org/10.1111/bioe.12786.

78. Blasimme A. Regenerative Medicine, Unproven Therapies and the Framing of Clinical Risk. In: Extraordinary risks, Ordinary lives. Palgrave Macmillan; 2022. p. 91–117.

79. Sipp D, Caulfield T, Kaye J, et al. Marketing of unproven stem cell-based interventions: A call to action. Sci Transl Med 2017;9(397). https://doi.org/10.1126/scitranslmed.aag0426.

80. Boardman F. Human genome editing and the identity politics of genetic disability. J Community Genet 2020;11(2):125–7. https://doi.org/10.1007/s12687-019-00437-4.

81. Parens E, Asch A. Disability rights critique of prenatal genetic testing: Reflections and recommendations. Ment Retard Dev Disabil Res Rev 2003;9(December 2002):40–7. https://doi.org/10.1002/mrdd.10056.

82. Elliott K, Ahlawat N, Beckman ES, et al. I wouldn't want anything that would change who he is. The relationship between perceptions of identity and attitudes towards hypothetical gene-editing in parents of children with autosomal aneuploidies. SSM - Qualitative Research in Health 2022;100151. https://doi.org/10.1016/j.ssmqr.2022.100151.

83. Snure Beckman E, Deuitch N, Michie M, et al. Attitudes toward hypothetical uses of gene-editing technologies in parents of people with autosomal aneuploidies. CRISPR j 2019;2(5):324–30. https://doi.org/10.1089/crispr.2019.0021.

84. Booth A, Bonham V, Porteus M, et al. Treatment decision-making in sickle cell disease patients. J Community Genet 2022;13(1):143–51. https://doi.org/10.1007/s12687-021-00562-z.

85. Hoffman-Andrews L, Mazzoni R, Pacione M, et al. Attitudes of people with inherited retinal conditions toward gene editing technology. Mol Genet Genomic Med 2019;7(7):e00803. https://doi.org/10.1002/mgg3.803.

86. Michie M, Allyse M. Gene modification therapies: views of parents of people with Down syndrome. Genet Med 2018. https://doi.org/10.1038/s41436-018-0077-6.

87. Wojcik MH, Schwartz TS, Yamin I, et al. Genetic disorders and mortality in infancy and early childhood: delayed diagnoses and missed opportunities. Genet Med 2018;20(11):1396–404. https://doi.org/10.1038/gim.2018.17.

88. Willig LK, Petrikin JE, Smith LD, et al. Whole-genome sequencing for identification of Mendelian disorders in critically ill infants: A retrospective analysis of diagnostic and clinical findings. Lancet Respir Med 2015;3(5):377–87. https://doi.org/10.1016/S2213-2600(15)00139-3.

89. Wojcik MH, D'Gama AM, Agrawal PB. A model to implement genomic medicine in the neonatal intensive care unit. J Perinatol 2022. https://doi.org/10.1038/s41372-022-01428-z.

90. Petrikin JE, Cakici JA, Clark MM, et al. The NSIGHT1-randomized controlled trial: rapid whole-genome sequencing for accelerated etiologic diagnosis in critically ill infants. NPJ Genom Med 2018;3:6. https://doi.org/10.1038/s41525-018-0045-8.

91. Kingsmore SF, Smith LD, Kunard CM, et al. A genome sequencing system for universal newborn screening, diagnosis, and precision medicine for severe genetic diseases. Am J Hum Genet 2022;109(9):1605–19. https://doi.org/10.1016/j.ajhg.2022.08.003.

92. French CE, Delon I, Dolling H, et al. Whole genome sequencing reveals that genetic conditions are frequent in intensively ill children. Intensive Care Med 2019; 45(5):627–36. https://doi.org/10.1007/s00134-019-05552-x.
93. Santoro JD, Bennett M. Ethics of End of Life Decisions in Pediatrics: A Narrative Review of the Roles of Caregivers, Shared Decision-Making, and Patient Centered Values. Behav Sci 2018;8(5). https://doi.org/10.3390/bs8050042.
94. Friebert S. Nondisclosure and emerging autonomy in a terminally ill teenager. Virtual Mentor 2010;12(7):522–9. https://doi.org/10.1001/virtualmentor.2010.12.7. ccas1-1007.
95. SECTION ON HOSPICE AND PALLIATIVE MEDICINE AND COMMITTEE ON HOSPITAL CARE. Pediatric Palliative Care and Hospice Care Commitments, Guidelines, and Recommendations. Pediatrics 2013;132(5):966–72. https://doi.org/10.1542/peds.2013-2731.

Essential Pieces to the Genetics Puzzle

Family History and Dysmorphology Exam

Allison Tam, MD

KEYWORDS

• Family history • Pedigree • Dysmorphology • Genetics evaluation

KEY POINTS

• Family history and physical exam findings are frequently the first clues that prompt primary care physicians to consider medical genetics evaluation.
• Pedigree facilitates the identification of classic Mendelian inheritance patterns from the family history.
• There is standardized nomenclature for human pedigree.
• It is important to consider observed physical features in the context of clinical history, family history, and the entire constellation of physical examination findings.
• There is standardized nomenclature for the description of physical features.

INTRODUCTION

While individual genetic diagnoses are rare, aggregate health conditions that have a genetic component are common. Mendelian conditions are estimated to be present in 8% of live births.[1] Family history and physical exam findings are frequently the first clues that prompt medical providers to consider clinical genetics evaluation. Family history is information on health history of an individual's biological relatives.[2] Family history has broad clinical utility. It allows assessment for the baseline likelihoods of genetic conditions given specific clinical findings.[1] In addition to its relevance for genetic conditions with Mendelian inheritance, family history can demonstrate major risk factors for several chronic diseases including cardiovascular disease, diabetes, osteoporosis, asthma and psychiatric disorders.[2] Taking a family history is inexpensive and does not require any invasive procedure. A good physical exam, which includes the detection and accurate description of dysmorphic features, is also key to prompting the consideration of Mendelian genetic conditions. Dysmorphology was initially described by Dr. David Smith in 1966 as the "study of, or general subject of, abnormal

Department of Pediatrics, University of California San Francisco, 550 16th Street, 4th Floor, San Francisco, CA 94143, USA
E-mail address: Allison.tam@ucsf.edu

Pediatr Clin N Am 70 (2023) 1047–1056
https://doi.org/10.1016/j.pcl.2023.05.012
0031-3955/23/© 2023 Elsevier Inc. All rights reserved.

development of tissue form."[3] It has since become a discipline that focuses on variations in physical features. Some physical features individually or in constellation can be suggestive of specific genetic disorders. Similar to family history, dysmorphology exam is inexpensive and easy to perform in the clinic. Despite advances in available technology including genomic sequencing and facial recognition software, it remains essential to systematically evaluate a patient, which includes taking an appropriate history and conduct a physical examination, to help generate differential diagnosis and plan in a clinical genetics evaluation. The goal of this article is to provide an overview of family history and dysmorphology exam, and their relevance for the clinical genetics evaluation.

DISCUSSION
Family History

A complete family history often contains health information on at least 3 generations of family members from both sides of the parents of the patient.[2,4] This can include children, siblings, and parents who are first-degree relatives; aunts, uncles, and grandparents who are second-degree relatives, and first cousins who are third-degree relatives. Some of the key health and demographic information that is helpful to document in a family history includes age at the time the pedigree was obtained, age at death and cause of death, miscarriages, major health conditions and the age at diagnosis, country of ancestral origin for both sets of grandparents if known, and whether a person's parents are closely related.[2] Depending on the clinical indication, environmental and occupational exposures may be relevant as well. The date on which the information was collected, the person who provided the information, and the person who obtained the information should ideally be noted.[4] Certain genetic conditions are more common in some populations than others, therefore, information on the country of ancestral origin can be helpful. It is also helpful in the context of gene variant interpretation. Most of the genetic population studies have focused on individuals of European ancestry. Individuals from underrepresented population may be more likely to have a genetic variant of uncertain significance than individuals of European ancestry.[5] In addition, offspring of parents who are closely related are at slightly increased risk of having a recessive disorder. Therefore, noting whether parents are consanguineous is helpful when obtaining family history.

Family history can be displayed graphically in the form of a pedigree. **Fig. 1** is an example of a pedigree which demonstrates some of the commonly used nomenclature. There is standardized nomenclature for human pedigree, and most refer to the expert opinions from the "Recommendations for human standardized pedigree nomenclature" initially published in 1995, and with updated recommendations published in 2008.[6,7] Bennett and colleagues published a focused revision in 2022 of the pedigree nomenclature to provide the clarification of the use of symbols and language in the description of the distinction between sex and gender.[8] The goal is to ensure safe and inclusive practice. In this revision, sex is defined by morphology or biology (phenotype, karyotype, and so forth), and gender refers to social constructions of roles, behaviors, expressions, and identities of men, women, boys, girls, and gender diverse people.[8] The pedigree symbols include squares, circles, and diamonds. They represent gender, and not sex assigned at birth.[8] A square represents an individual who identifies as man or boy. A circle represents an individual who identifies as woman or girl. A diamond represents gender not known, gender not specified, gender non-binary, or gender diverse.[8] Information that may be placed below the symbol includes the age of the individual, or one can note the year of birth (eg, b.1960) and/or

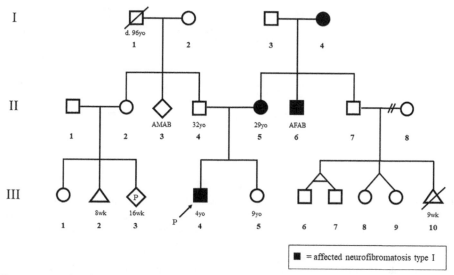

Fig. 1. Example of a pedigree to illustrate pedigree nomenclature based on recommendations published by Bennett and colleagues in 2022.[8] I-1 is deceased, with notation "d. 96yo" to represent age of death. Line connecting between I-1 and I-2 indicates relationship. A break between the line connecting between II-7 and II-8 indicates the relationship no longer exists. II-3 who was assigned male at birth identifies as gender non-binary, this is represented by diamond symbol and the notation "AMAB." III-6 who was assigned female at birth identifies as man, this is represented by a square symbol and the notation "AFAB." III-2 indicates spontaneous abortion at 8 weeks gestational age. III-3 indicates pregnancy with unknown fetal sex and 16 weeks gestational age. III-6 and III-7 are monozygotic twins. III-8 and III-9 are dizygotic twins. III-10 indicates the termination of pregnancy at 9 weeks of gestational age. I-4 is the proband, which is represented with arrow pointed at the symbol. Shaded symbol represents clinically affected individuals, in this pedigree I-4, II-5, II-6, and III-4 are affected. Shading should be defined, and the legend for this pedigree is in the left lower corner.

year of death (eg, d. 2021), and notation that indicates the assigned sex at birth for an individual whose gender identity or gender expression does not align with the sex they were assigned a birth (ie, AFAB = Assigned Female at Birth, AMAB = Assigned Male At Birth, UAAB = Unassigned At Birth).[8] In addition, other information that may be placed below the symbol can also include relevant evaluation results including gene variant or karyotype and pedigree number (eg, I-1, II-1, II-2) particularly if used in publication.[8] Bennett and colleagues have updated recommendation on carrier status depiction. In response to the increased recognition that heterozygous carriers of many X-linked recessive conditions may have clinical manifestations, the single dot that previously was used to represent carrier status is no longer recommended in the focused revision by Bennett and colleagues.[8] The authors recommended that the symbol be divided and a unique fill pattern be provided for the subsection to represent the different carrier results and/or clinical manifestations.[8] The fill patterns are explained in the pedigree legend.[8]

One main advantage of having family history presented in the form of pedigree is to facilitate the identification of classic Mendelian inheritance patterns, such as autosomal dominant, autosomal recessive, and X-linked recessive inheritance patterns. **Fig. 2** shows examples of pedigrees that suggest different inheritance patterns. Characteristics of autosomal dominant inheritance pattern includes the condition can be

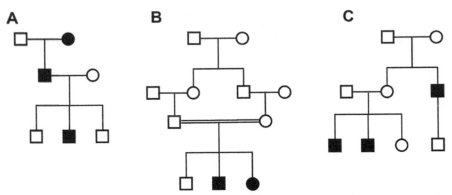

Fig. 2. Example of pedigrees suggestive of autosomal dominant, autosomal recessive, and X-linked recessive inheritance patterns. (*A*) Shows an autosomal dominant inheritance pattern: affected individuals in successive generations, male and female family members are equally likely to be affected, and there can be male-to-male transmission. (*B*) Shows an autosomal recessive inheritance pattern: affected individuals often have unaffected parents, multiple siblings affected, male and female family members are equally likely to be affected. In addition, offspring of parents who are closely related, indicated by the double line, are at slightly increased risk of having a recessive disorder. (*C*) Shows an X-linked recessive inheritance pattern: males are primarily affected in the family, carrier female may be unaffected or mildly affected, no male-to-male transmission, affected males transmit the gene variant to all daughters but not to any of their sons.

present in individuals in successive generations, male and female family members are equally likely to be affected and there is male-to-male transmission. However, it is possible for an individual to be affected by an autosomal dominant disorder with no family history, in which the genetic defect is typically found to be *de novo* in that individual. Characteristic of an autosomal recessive inheritance pattern includes affected individuals often have unaffected parents, multiple siblings affected, and male and female family members are equally likely to be affected. Offspring of consanguineous parents are at slightly increased risk of having an autosomal recessive disorder. Characteristics of X-linked recessive inheritance pattern includes males are primarily affected in the family, carrier females may be unaffected or mildly affected, no male-to-male transmission, affected males transmit the gene variant to all daughters but not to any of their sons. In addition to facilitating the identification of inheritance patterns, having a pedigree also helps in the identification of other family members who might be at risk for a genetic condition if a genetic diagnosis is known in at least one individual. For example, if the proband was found to have Duchenne muscular dystrophy and has a hemizygous *DMD* pathogenic variant, then we can use the pedigree to more easily identify which family members might be at risk based on the knowledge that this is an X-linked condition.

There may not be adequate time allowed to obtain a comprehensive, three-generation family history in the primary care setting. Targeted family history focusing on specific disorders relevant to presenting symptom, or tailored family history focusing on a range of disorders relevant to child's age-based health, may be appropriate during acute care and routine well-child clinic visits.[2] If there are red flags identified, clinicians may consider obtaining a comprehensive three-generation family history, performing additional studies and/or initiating referral to genetics specialists. Therefore, it is important to recognize red flags. Red flags may include family history of a Mendelian genetic condition, multiple relatives on the same side of the family that are affected with the same disorder (two or more closely related relatives on the same side of the family), a person with more than one major health condition or medical event, earlier-than-expected age at onset of disease, sudden death without a clear cause, medical problems in the offspring of consanguineous parents, and unusual presentation of the condition.[4]

A positive family history may prompt more specific genetic evaluation for a patient. If there is a family history of a family member with known genetic condition, it is generally the preferred approach to test the person who is most likely to have a positive result with genetic testing. If that person has a positive test, then the result can guide targeted, cascade testing for other relatives at risk. A pedigree can be a clear representation of the family history to help determine which family members should be tested. While a negative family history could also be valuable information, it does not completely exclude the possibility of a Mendelian genetic disorder. For example, an individual might have a genetic condition that is not inherited from either parent and have a *de novo*, genetic defect. One should also consider the possibility of incomplete penetrance and variable expressivity of a Mendelian condition even among affected members from the same family.

Family history can be extremely useful, but it relies on the collected information to be reliable and accurate. In a pediatric clinic setting, the historian providing the family history is often one or both parents. However, the historian may also be other family members, adoptive parents, or foster parents. The availability and accuracy of family history may differ depending on the historian. It is also important to note that family history may change through time, in other words it is dynamic. It is helpful to take note of the date the family history is obtained, and family history may need to be updated from time to time. Potential challenges in obtaining family history includes time limitation during the clinic visit, absence of available family history for example, in cases which the patient was adopted, and historian(s) "misinterpret, fail to disclose or simply be unaware of information."[2] Health care providers should be mindful of these challenges when assessing reported family history. At the same time, family history can be a sensitive topic. Sharing very personal information such as death or serious medical condition of relatives can be difficult. Clinicians should always be sensitive and respectful when obtaining family history.

Dysmorphology

Physical features can differ in number, size, placement, and shape. Dysmorphic features refer to the structural developmental that is out of the ordinary.[9] There are few major categories of anomalies, including malformations, disruptions, deformations, and dysplasias.

- A malformation is a morphological defect of an organ, part of an organ, or a larger region of the body resulting from an intrinsically abnormal developmental process.[10]
- A disruption is a morphological defect of an organ, part of an organ, or a larger region of the body resulting from the extrinsic breakdown of, or an interference with, an originally normal developmental process.[10]
- A deformation is an abnormal form, shape, or position of a part of the body caused by mechanical forces.[10]
- A dysplasia is an abnormal organization of cells into tissue(s) and its morphologic result(s).[10]

Understanding the differences between these anomalies can provide insight into an assessment of the underlying etiology for the anomaly. Genetic etiology is more likely if the anomaly is related to malformation or dysplasia. On the other hand, environmental etiology is more likely if the anomaly is related to disruption or deformation.[1]

Clinician should approach the physical examination in an objective manner.[9] It is often informative to assess height, weight, and head circumference, followed by a systematic examination of structure.[9] It is important to consider that there is normal variation in physical features in the population. Being able to describe a feature in detail using consistent terminology is important for both clinical and research purposes. One of the most used resources for the standardized nomenclature for physical feature descriptions is The Elements of Morphology. It is available online free of charge (http://elementsofmorphology.nih.gov).[11] There are also various key publications on morphologic variants of the human body.[12–18] **Table 1** lists examples of standardized terms used to describe human morphology. Specific measurements can sometimes be helpful in more accurately documenting the size of a physical feature and more

Table 1
Examples of terms used to describe human morphology

Head	Nose	Hands
Macrocephaly	Low hanging columella	Clinodactyly
Microcephaly	Anteverted nares	Prominent digit pad
Brachycephaly	Wide nasal base	Cutaneous syndactyly of fingers
Low anterior hairline	Depressed nasal bridge	Overlapping fingers
Sparse scalp hair		Short finger
		Small hand
Face	*Philtrum*	Split hand
Coarse face	Long philtrum	Single transverse palmer crease
Long face	Smooth philtrum	Small nail
Triangular face		
Frontal bossing	*Lip*	*Feet*
Midface retrusion	Lip pit	Postaxial polydactyly of foot
Micrognathia	Tented vermilion of the upper lip	Preaxial polydactyly of foot
Tall chin	Thin vermilion of the upper lip	Broad hallux
		Pes planus
Neck	*Mouth*	Pes cavus
Neck webbing	Downturned corners of mouth	
Long neck	Wide mouth	*Trunk*
	Single maxillary central incisor	Pectus excavatum
Ear	Dental crowding	Pectus carinatum
Cupped ear	Oligodontia	Supernumerary nipple
Low-set ear	High palate	Wide-spaced nipple
Protruding ear	Widely spaced teeth	
Overfolded helix	Large tongue	
Uplifted lobe	Protruding tongue	
Microtia	Cleft uvula	
Preauricular pit		
Preauricular tag		

objectively distinguish the variation from expected ranges. For example, it can be challenging to subjectively determine that an individual's palpebral fissures are short. The length of palpebral fissure can be determined objectively by measuring the distance between the medial and lateral aspects of the eyelids, or canthi, and short palpebral fissure refers to the palpebral fissure length more than two standard deviation below the mean for age.[13] Determination of the presence of short palpebral fissures can be crucial, for example, if fetal alcohol spectrum disorders are being considered. References that are helpful in body part measurement have been provided.[19,20] Documenting dysmorphic features accurately may allow better assessment of potential differential diagnosis for an individual with a clinical presentation suggestive of an underlying genetic syndrome.

Physical features may have varying clinical significance or no clinical significance. For example, fifth finger clinodactyly can be observed in isolation as a normal variation, or as part of constellation of physical features in certain symptoms such as Down syndrome. Some physical features are relatively common in certain populations compared to the others. For example, thick vermillion borders of the lips and broad nasal bridge are relatively common in African populations, but much less common in white populations.[21] In essence, it important to consider observed physical features in the context of clinical history, family history and the entire physical examination findings. The identified patterns may sometimes suggest specific genetic or environmental etiologies. There are some terms that are used to describe various types of anomaly patterns. For example,.

- A developmental field defect is a pattern of anomalies derived from the disturbance of a single developmental field.[10]
- A sequence is a pattern of multiple anomalies derived from a single known or presumed previous anomaly or mechanical factor.[10]
- A syndrome is a pattern of multiple anomalies thought to be pathogenetically related and not known to represent a single sequence or developmental field defect.[10]
- An association is a nonrandom occurrence in 2 or more individuals of multiple anomalies not known to be a developmental field defect, a sequence, or a syndrome.[10]

Recognition of patterns may rely on one's clinical knowledge and experience, but there are also resources that are available to facilitate the process. For example, clinical findings include physical features can be entered in the search for genetic conditions through the Online Mendelian Inheritance in Man (OMIM ; Johns Hopkins University, Baltimore, MD) database.[22] There are also resources such as the Face2-Gene smartphone application which uses automated facial feature analysis to help in the generation of genetic differential diagnosis.[1,23]

The main objective of the identification and accurate description of dysmorphic features is to allow the recognition of patterns, and ultimately help in reaching the clinical diagnoses for our patients. Consider a case example in which the clinician performs physical examination on a neonate and noted the following findings: cloverleaf skull, midface retrusion, downslanted palpebral fissures, proptosis, high palate, bilateral cutaneous syndactyly of the fingers, bilateral cutaneous syndactyly of the toes, and broad distal hallux. The findings from dysmorphology examination suggest high likelihood of a genetic etiology. Using standardized terminology, the clinician can communicate these findings with other clinicians including a medical genetics specialist. One may immediately consider the genetic diagnosis of Apert syndrome given the constellation of physical features.[24] Suspicion for Apert syndrome may in turn guide the decision on further studies such as *FGFR2* gene sequencing, and immediate management such as attention to potential airway obstruction that is indicated for the neonate.

Lastly, genetic syndromes may present differently across different population groups. There has been increased recognition that many of the medical textbooks and much of the clinical genetics literature are focused on individuals of Northern European descent, despite the fact that genetic syndromes affect people globally.[21] This has led to the rise in the characterization of genetic syndromes in diverse population in the medical literature.[21] It is important for clinicians to recognize that some of the classic genetic syndromes that are described in medical literature may show variation in dysmorphic facial features among affected individuals of different ancestry. For example, facial features in Africans with 22q11.2 deletion syndrome differ from those in whites. Nasal anomaly is one of the classic features noted in individuals of European ancestry with 22q11.2; however, only 15% to 40% of individuals of African descent had nasal deformity.[21] Interestingly, Kruszka and colleagues explored the use of facial analysis technology as an objective assessment of dysmorphic features, in addition to physical exam in diverse populations. The authors found that facial analysis technology is accurate in diagnosing genetic syndrome in diverse populations.[21] Nonetheless, it is important for medical and research communities to ensure the characterization of genetic syndromes in diverse population when possible.

SUMMARY

Identification of key information from family history and specific dysmorphic features are often the first clues that suggest potential genetic diagnoses, leading to further genetic evaluation. Obtaining family history and observing physical features are both inexpensive and easy to perform in the pediatric clinics. Using standardized nomenclature for both the pedigree and description of physical features is important for clinical documentation; furthermore, it is helpful in research and publication. Family history and dysmorphic features contribute significantly to the genetic differential diagnosis, therefore they are essential to the consideration of subsequent diagnostic work-up, including genetic testing.

CLINICS CARE POINTS

- Family history can be displayed graphically in the form of a pedigree.

- There is standardized nomenclature for human pedigrees.

- Important red flags from family history that may prompt further genetic evaluation may include family history of a Mendelian genetic condition, multiple relatives on the same side of the family affected with the same disorder (two or more closely related relatives on the same side of the family), and earlier-than-expected age at onset of disease.

- There is standardized nomenclature for the description of variation in physical features.

- Some of the classic genetic syndromes that are described in medical literature may have different dysmorphic facial features among affected individuals of different ancestry.

DISCLOSURE

Nothing to disclose.

REFERENCES

1. Kim AY, Bodurtha JN. Dysmorphology. Pediatr Rev 2019;40(12):609–18. https://doi.org/10.1542/PIR.2018-0331.
2. Tarini BA, McInerney JD. Family history in primary care pediatrics. Pediatrics 2013;132(Suppl 3). https://doi.org/10.1542/PEDS.2013-1032D.
3. Smith DW. Dysmorphology (teratology). J Pediatr 1966;69(6):1150–69. https://doi.org/10.1016/S0022-3476(66)80311-6.
4. Bennett RL. Family Health History: The First Genetic Test in Precision Medicine. Med Clin North Am 2019;103(6):957–66. https://doi.org/10.1016/J.MCNA.2019.06.002.
5. Popejoy AB, Fullerton SM. Genomics is failing on diversity. Nature 2016;538(7624):161–4. https://doi.org/10.1038/538161A.
6. Bennett RL, French KS, Resta RG, et al, Doyle DL. Standardized human pedigree nomenclature: update and assessment of the recommendations of the National Society of Genetic Counselors. J Genet Counsel 2008;17(5):424–33. https://doi.org/10.1007/S10897-008-9169-9.
7. Bennett RL, Steinhaus KA, Uhrich SB, et al. Recommendations for standardized human pedigree nomenclature. J Genet Counsel 1995;4(4):267–79. https://doi.org/10.1007/BF01408073.
8. Bennett RL, French KS, Resta RG, et al. Practice resource-focused revision: Standardized pedigree nomenclature update centered on sex and gender inclusivity: A practice resource of the National Society of Genetic Counselors. J Genet Counsel 2022. https://doi.org/10.1002/JGC4.1621.
9. Genetics AC on. Medical Genetics in Pediatric Practice. Medical Genetics in Pediatric Practice 2013. https://doi.org/10.1542/9781581104974.
10. Spranger J, Benirschke K, Hall JG, et al. Errors of morphogenesis: concepts and terms. Recommendations of an international working group. J Pediatr 1982;100(1):160–5. https://doi.org/10.1016/S0022-3476(82)80261-8.
11. Elements of Morphology: Human Malformation Terminology. Available at: https://elementsofmorphology.nih.gov/index.cgi. Accessed September 24, 2022.
12. Allanson JE, Biesecker LG, Carey JC, et al. Elements of morphology: introduction. Am J Med Genet 2009;149A(1):2–5. https://doi.org/10.1002/AJMG.A.32601.
13. Hall BD, Graham JM, Cassidy SB, et al. Elements of morphology: standard terminology for the periorbital region. Am J Med Genet 2009;149A(1):29–39. https://doi.org/10.1002/AJMG.A.32597.
14. Hennekam RCM, Cormier-Daire V, Hall JG, et al. Elements of morphology: Standard terminology for the nose and philtrum. Am J Med Genet 2009;149(1):61–76. https://doi.org/10.1002/ajmg.a.32600.
15. Allanson JE, Cunniff C, Eugene Hoyme H, et al. Elements of morphology: Standard terminology for the head and face. Am J Med Genet 2009;149(1):6–28. https://doi.org/10.1002/ajmg.a.32612.
16. Carey JC, Cohen MM, Curry CJR, et al. Elements of morphology: standard terminology for the lips, mouth, and oral region. Am J Med Genet 2009;149A(1):77–92. https://doi.org/10.1002/AJMG.A.32602.
17. Hunter A, Frias JL, Gillessen-Kaesbach G, et al. Elements of morphology: standard terminology for the ear. Am J Med Genet 2009;149A(1):40–60. https://doi.org/10.1002/AJMG.A.32599.
18. Biesecker LG, Aase JM, Clericuzio C, et al. Elements of morphology: standard terminology for the hands and feet. Am J Med Genet 2009;149A(1):93–127. https://doi.org/10.1002/AJMG.A.32596.

19. Gripp KW, Slavotinek AM, Hall JG, et al. Handbook of Physical Measurements. Handbook of Physical Measurements 2013. https://doi.org/10.1093/MED/9780199935710.001.0001.

20. Jones K, Jones M, Campo M del. Smith's Recognizable Patterns of Human Malformation.; 2013. Available at: https://books.google.com/books?hl=en&lr=&id=idyBAAAAQBAJ&oi=fnd&pg=PP1&ots=ELRLbk7g0t&sig=eHiaWl_CyoUAzYxUrhw1IONrt0E. Accessed September 22, 2022.

21. Kruszka P, Tekendo-Ngongang C, Muenke M. Diversity and dysmorphology. Curr Opin Pediatr 2019;31(6):702–7. https://doi.org/10.1097/MOP.0000000000000816.

22. OMIM. Available at: https://www.omim.org/. Accessed September 27, 2022.

23. Face2Gene. Available at: https://www.face2gene.com/. Accessed September 27, 2022.

24. Wilkie AOM, Slaney SF, Oldridge M, et al. Apert syndrome results from localized mutations of FGFR2 and is allelic with Crouzon syndrome. Nat Genet 1995;9(2). https://doi.org/10.1038/ng0295-165.

UNITED STATES POSTAL SERVICE ® Statement of Ownership, Management, and Circulation (All Periodicals Publications Except Requester Publications)

1. Publication Title	2. Publication Number	3. Filing Date
PEDIATRIC CLINICS OF NORTH AMERICA	424 – 66	9/18/2023

4. Issue Frequency	5. Number of Issues Published Annually	6. Annual Subscription Price
FEB, APR, JUN, AUG, OCT, DEC	6	$279.00

7. Complete Mailing Address of Known Office of Publication (Not printer) (Street, city, county, state, and ZIP+4®)

ELSEVIER INC.
230 Park Avenue, Suite 800
New York, NY 10169

Contact Person
Malathi Samayan

Telephone (Include area code)
91-44-4299-4507

8. Complete Mailing Address of Headquarters or General Business Office of Publisher (Not printer)

ELSEVIER INC.
230 Park Avenue, Suite 800
New York, NY 10169

9. Full Names and Complete Mailing Addresses of Publisher, Editor, and Managing Editor (Do not leave blank)

Publisher (Name and complete mailing address)

Dolores Meloni, ELSEVIER INC.
1600 JOHN F KENNEDY BLVD. SUITE 1600
PHILADELPHIA, PA 19103-2899

Editor (Name and complete mailing address)

KERRY HOLLAND, ELSEVIER INC.
1600 JOHN F KENNEDY BLVD. SUITE 1600
PHILADELPHIA, PA 19103-2899

Managing Editor (Name and complete mailing address)

PATRICK MANLEY, ELSEVIER INC.
1600 JOHN F KENNEDY BLVD. SUITE 1600
PHILADELPHIA, PA 19103-2899

10. Owner (Do not leave blank. If the publication is owned by a corporation, give the name and address of the corporation immediately followed by the names and addresses of all stockholders owning or holding 1 percent or more of the total amount of stock. If not owned by a corporation, give the names and addresses of the individual owners. If owned by a partnership or other unincorporated firm, give its name and address as well as those of each individual owner. If the publication is published by a nonprofit organization, give its name and address.)

Full Name	Complete Mailing Address
WHOLLY OWNED SUBSIDIARY OF REED/ELSEVIER, US HOLDINGS	1600 JOHN F KENNEDY BLVD, SUITE 1600 PHILADELPHIA, PA 19103-2899

11. Known Bondholders, Mortgagees, and Other Security Holders Owning or Holding 1 Percent or More of Total Amount of Bonds, Mortgages, or Other Securities. If none, check box ▶ ☐ None

Full Name	Complete Mailing Address
N/A	

12. Tax Status (For completion by nonprofit organizations authorized to mail at nonprofit rates) (Check one)
The purpose, function, and nonprofit status of this organization and the exempt status for federal income tax purposes:
☒ Has Not Changed During Preceding 12 Months
☐ Has Changed During Preceding 12 Months (Publisher must submit explanation of change with this statement)

PS Form **3526**, July 2014 [Page 1 of 4 (see instructions page 4)] PSN: 7530-01-000-9931 PRIVACY NOTICE: See our privacy policy on www.usps.com.

---

13. Publication Title	14. Issue Date for Circulation Data Below
PEDIATRIC CLINICS OF NORTH AMERICA	AUGUST 2023

15. Extent and Nature of Circulation		Average No. Copies Each Issue During Preceding 12 Months	No. Copies of Single Issue Published Nearest to Filing Date
a. Total Number of Copies (Net press run)		340	339
b. Paid Circulation (By Mail and Outside the Mail)	(1) Mailed Outside-County Paid Subscriptions Stated on PS Form 3541 (Include paid distribution above nominal rate, advertiser's proof copies, and exchange copies)	188	186
	(2) Mailed In-County Paid Subscriptions Stated on PS Form 3541 (Include paid distribution above nominal rate, advertiser's proof copies, and exchange copies)	0	0
	(3) Paid Distribution Outside the Mails Including Sales Through Dealers and Carriers, Street Vendors, Counter Sales, and Other Paid Distribution Outside USPS®	135	127
	(4) Paid Distribution by Other Classes of Mail Through the USPS (e.g., First-Class Mail®)	12	22
c. Total Paid Distribution (Sum of 15b (1), (2), (3), and (4))	▶	335	335
d. Free or Nominal Rate Distribution (By Mail and Outside the Mail)	(1) Free or Nominal Rate Outside-County Copies included on PS Form 3541	4	4
	(2) Free or Nominal Rate In-County Copies Included on PS Form 3541	0	0
	(3) Free or Nominal Rate Copies Mailed at Other Classes Through the USPS (e.g., First-Class Mail)	0	0
	(4) Free or Nominal Rate Distribution Outside the Mail (Carriers or other means)	1	0
e. Total Free or Nominal Rate Distribution (Sum of 15d (1), (2), (3) and (4))	▶	5	4
f. Total Distribution (Sum of 15c and 15e)	▶	340	339
g. Copies not Distributed (See Instructions to Publishers #4 (page #3))	▶	0	0
h. Total (Sum of 15f and g)	▶	340	339
i. Percent Paid (15c divided by 15f times 100)		98.53%	98.82%

* If you are claiming electronic copies, go to line 16 on page 3. If you are not claiming electronic copies, skip to line 17 on page 3.

16. Electronic Copy Circulation		Average No. Copies Each Issue During Preceding 12 Months	No. Copies of Single Issue Published Nearest to Filing Date
a. Paid Electronic Copies	▶		
b. Total Paid Print Copies (Line 15c) + Paid Electronic Copies (Line 16a)	▶		
c. Total Print Distribution (Line 15f) + Paid Electronic Copies (Line 16a)	▶		
d. Percent Paid (Both Print & Electronic Copies) (16b divided by 16c × 100)	▶		

☒ I certify that 50% of all my distributed copies (electronic and print) are paid above a nominal price.

17. Publication of Statement of Ownership

☒ If the publication is a general publication, publication of this statement is required. Will be printed in the OCTOBER 2023 issue of this publication. ☐ Publication not required.

18. Signature and Title of Editor, Publisher, Business Manager, or Owner

Malathi Samayan — Distribution Controller

Malathi Samayan - Distribution Controller

Date 9/18/2023

I certify that all information furnished on this form is true and complete. I understand that anyone who furnishes false or misleading information on this form or who omits material or information requested on the form may be subject to criminal sanctions (including fines and imprisonment) and/or civil sanctions (including civil penalties).

PS Form **3526**, July 2014 (Page 2 of 4)

PRIVACY NOTICE: See our privacy policy on www.usps.com

Moving?

Make sure your subscription moves with you!

To notify us of your new address, find your **Clinics Account Number** (located on your mailing label above your name), and contact customer service at:

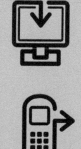

Email: journalscustomerservice-usa@elsevier.com

800-654-2452 (subscribers in the U.S. & Canada)
314-447-8871 (subscribers outside of the U.S. & Canada)

Fax number: 314-447-8029

Elsevier Health Sciences Division
Subscription Customer Service
3251 Riverport Lane
Maryland Heights, MO 63043

ELSEVIER

Printed and bound by CPI Group (UK) Ltd, Croydon, CR0 4YY

03/10/2024

01040471-0020